D0172004

LIVING WELL

LIVING WELL

Robert Warren

Fount
An Imprint of HarperCollins*Publishers*

Fount is an imprint of
HarperCollins*Religious*
Part of HarperCollins*Publishers*
77–85 Fulham Palace Road, London W6 8JB

First published in Great Britain in 1998 by Fount
1 3 5 7 9 10 8 6 4 2

A catalogue record for this book is
available from the British Library

ISBN 0 00 628100 1

Printed and bound in Great Britain by
Caledonian International Book Manufacturing Ltd, Glasgow

THE BEATITUDES

Blessed are the poor in spirit,
for theirs is the kingdom of heaven.
Blessed are those who mourn, for they will be comforted.
Blessed are the meek, for they will inherit the earth.
Blessed are those who hunger and thirst for righteousness,
for they will be filled.
Blessed are the merciful, for they will receive mercy.
Blessed are the pure in heart, for they will see God.
Blessed are the peacemakers,
for they will be called children of God.
Blessed are those who are persecuted for righteousness' sake,
for theirs is the kingdom of heaven.

CONTENTS

Part Four: Living differently

FOREWORD

Few other people are as well placed as Robert Warren to reflect on the mission of the Church of England today. His outstanding parochial ministry at St Thomas Crookes in Sheffield coupled, more recently, with his work as the National Officer for Evangelism, have given him experiences at both local and national levels that few can rival. Moreover his seminal work on church planting and building missionary congregations has greatly benefited many parishes up and down the country.

But in this new book he shares with us another of his passions – Jesus' teaching on the way we should live our lives as we find it summarized in his Beatitudes. Go into many of our older churches and you will still find inscribed, either on the walls or on wooden panels, both the Ten Commandments and the Beatitudes. Today, as he rightly points out, the Church still acknowledges the significance of the former but has tended to lose sight of the foundational significance of the latter, both for personal and community living.

Yet for many centuries it was those first few verses in Matthew 5 that provided the bedrock of Christian ethical instruction and it is this perspective that he is seeking to recapture, albeit in a very changed cultural situation. Not being content to leave them as a series of impossible demands, or so 'other-worldly' that they have no relevance to day to day living, he seeks out their meaning for today and offers practical help in applying them to our lives.

Like his other recent books, this one is intended to lead to change. His helpful meditations and reflections will be of equal value to individuals or small groups. In either case it is a book to take slowly as it needs time for prayer, stillness and serious thought between every chapter; for only through those will we discover something more of what it means to 'live well'.

I am delighted that Robert accepted my invitation to write my 1999 Lent Book and I warmly commend it to you.

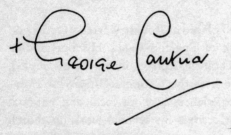

Archbishop of Canterbury

INTRODUCTION

THE SEARCH IS ON

What an amazing world we live in. A world of the Internet and the terrorist, of the atom and abortion, of chips and the microchip, of keyhole surgery and Ecstasy tablets. It is an amazing, fast-changing world full of wonder, threat and opportunity; both comfortable and confusing. It is not a world that is easy to live in, though few of us would opt to live in any other period of history. We are glad to be living on this side of the invention of anaesthetics and electricity.

Many things contribute to this confusion. The way that change is taking place and the speed with which it is happening, has a great impact on us. Gone are the days of settled, stable communities, of families living within walking distance of each other. Gone are the old familiar social patterns. As someone has put it, in today's informal culture you really have to get to know someone quite well before you find out their surname!

The familiar landmarks, whether the corner shop, or the roads, the hedgerows and skylines, are changing all the time. Not only that, the goalposts have moved socially. We are not sure whether to ask someone if they are married or if they have a partner, and if we ask the latter we are then not sure which sex the person is.

I heard recently of two miners who returned after several years to the site of the pit at which they had spent their working lives. They were involved in a furious argument about whether the entrance to the mine shaft was 'over here' or 'over there'. What made the answer so difficult was that the mine had gone, the whole place had been landscaped. They were standing in the middle of a completely featureless area covering several acres. No wonder they could not find their bearings. And so say all of us! We find it difficult to get our bearings in a culture that has largely abandoned social roles and social norms and inherited ways of doing things.

Not that we can put the clock back. The only way out is through. We have to press on into a new order of reality. Which is why the search is on; but for what?

THE SEARCH FOR VALUES

Many things hold cultures and communities together, not least the power that the few have had over the many. That power has often been expressed through a controlling culture that demands certain behaviours of us all. Hence, for example, the power of respectability a century ago which necessitated the unmarried mother leaving the district and having her child where she was not known – 'for the good name of the family'. Many of these controlling, and often hypocritical, ways have gone. But the tide has also swept away many good and familiar social patterns of knowing, caring and simple awareness of the needs of those around us.

Behind those outward forms of behaviour lay values on which the social patterns were built. Not everything was good, but what those stronger patterns did achieve was a degree of social cohesion. Without shared values it is difficult for people to live together, unless every new action is to be negotiated from scratch.

That is a time-consuming process that would take most of us more than a lifetime.

Hence the search for values that might bind our society together. Schools are part of a national search for values in education. The European Community has a major values project seeking to discover the things that can hold the whole continent of Europe together. We know we cannot hold together as a community, nation, or culture, by force. It has to be by choice. Yet what might those choices be? What sort of values might hold us together?

As we move into the third millennium the Christian faith deserves exploring again to see if we can mine from it the values that could equip us for living in a post-industrial, post-colonial, post-modern, post-almost-everything world. Not that we are likely to find what we need for living in such a changed and changing world without reworking much of what we have inherited.

Any community experiencing loss of identity and purpose
and unable to reflect on its past cannot create a viable future.
Michael Crosby, *Spirituality of the Beatitudes*

A DOUBLE HINGE OF HISTORY

New beginnings are always moments of opportunity: in them we can look for ways to make a new start. Our present setting gives us a double reason for seeking to do just that.

First the very fact of the turn of the millennium is itself an opportunity for new beginnings. Marriage guidance counsellors advise that moving house is a dubious way of tackling marriage problems. More couples split up as a result of moving house than in relation to any other event. Yet it is possible to see that fact from another perspective. Moving house is the last desperate attempt to begin again. It is well intentioned, but too often does not bring the hoped-for solutions. We would do well to see the millennium in that light. Of itself, the change of date will not make us different. Yet, it contains within its striking symbolism the opportunity and potential to enable us to be different. Certainly, we shall need more than a change of the clocks to move us. That is why exploring the roots of the Christian heritage may well provide us with a route through to a new way of being human and of bringing cohesion to our culture.

Second, we are living in a period of profound change that also presents us with opportunities for a new beginning. Culture and society are like the continental plates beneath the earth's surface. They are always on the move – imperceptibly. For most of the time the change is not evident. But every now and again the next small move results in cataclysmic change, causing an earthquake or volcano. Then everything changes. The whole landscape is different. Like the miners in my story, we have great difficulty finding our bearings or knowing where we are. Today's world is going through just such a period of upheaval.

The Christian faith, and church, have a rich heritage at this very point. We have a vital role to play in sharing the insights from that tradition with the wider society. The danger is that we simply sit on, or retreat into, our rich past. Our heritage is rooted in the incarnate God – the One who loves the world, not just the church, and sends His people to share His life with that world. We have a responsibility to share the good news, which we have discovered, with others.

But before that, we need to let it speak to us afresh in the new situation we face. We cannot trot out the familiar truths as we heard them from the past and expect them to make sense in this changed world. Rather our need is to apply them, and express them in a way that makes connections today. We are not to repeat the truth unthinkingly, but rather to find in our day ways in which they can speak afresh to our world.

We are called to be physicians of that civilization
about which we dream, the civilization of love.

Pope Paul VI on New Year's Eve 1975,
exactly twenty-five years before the turn of the millennium

LIVING THE TRUTH

One of the great glories of the Christian faith is that it is intended not just to be studied or discussed, but lived. That is why the Judaeo-Christian scriptures are not primarily books on doctrine, but rather stories of how the revelation of God has made an impact and shaped the lives of those who have heard its message.

Which brings us to the central biblical text of this book, namely the Beatitudes. In them Jesus encapsulated the key characteristics of those who seek to follow His way. Here are the values by which followers of Christ are called to live. They also address the question of how that faith is to be given expression in daily living, so that the world around experiences the benefit of living in the wake of the practice of these values.

Our problem is that the Beatitudes themselves are a closed book to many of us. We are not really sure we know what they mean. And in so far as we do understand them, we are not sure that we agree with them. They seem to be something of a 'charter for wimps', well expressed in the rewriting of the fourth Beatitude as 'the meek shall inherit the earth – just as long as everybody else is happy with that arrangement!'

The aim of this book is to unlock the secrets of the Beatitudes; and to do so in such a way that they can shape the lives of Christian people, of churches, and thereby contribute to the renewal and 'holding together' of our whole society. For that to happen, Christians and churches need to be the first to take this 'medicine of immortality' to heart, and live it out.

The church must be the first sign of what it preaches.

Michael Crosby, *House of disciples*

OUR ROOTS IN THE BEATITUDES

One reason why the Beatitudes are such a closed book is that they have dropped out of significant visibility. In the early centuries they were one of the key texts for those being initiated into the faith – alongside the Lord's Prayer and the Creed. Those three texts helped newcomers to the faith to know what to believe (the Creed), how to pray (the Lord's Prayer) and how to live (the Beatitudes). Sadly, the Beatitudes are much less central to the life of the church than they used to be. No wonder we struggle to make sense of them. We often struggle to know what they are! Yet for much of the history of the church they have been the roots from which Christian spirituality, moral behaviour, and discipleship have been nourished and inspired. Here are some introductory points that can help to make sense of them.

Their setting

They come at the beginning of the Sermon on the Mount. That sermon, recorded in Matthew's gospel, has its parallel in Luke's gospel. It is the gathering together of much of the teaching ministry of Jesus. The Beatitudes describe the character of the 'child of the kingdom'. The rest of the sermon goes on to illustrate how those character traits, or values, work themselves out when faced with particular issues, such as conflict, materialism, personal relationships and religious practices.

Matthew's gospel is the most Jewish of the gospels and is shaped in five sections. Commentators see this as a conscious following of the five books of Moses, with the Beatitudes paralleling the Ten Commandments, and the Sermon on the Mount being the New Testament's equivalent of the full 'law' revealed to Moses.

Their shape

There is a wonderful beauty, order and rhythm in these Beatitudes. Each one begins with the assurance of God's blessing. 'Blessed' means that God's favour and goodness is upon such a person. This blessing involved the outpouring of God's love, affirmation, support, help and generosity on the one who is 'blessed'.

The heart of each Beatitude is a kingdom-characteristic, trait or value, which Jesus says is foundational to living as a child of the heavenly Father. They are surprising values since neither the culture of his day, nor ours, saw these things as in any sense 'blessed'. They are contrary to all natural perspectives on life. We would be more inclined to say not, 'Blessed are those who ...', but rather, 'You are in real trouble if you ... are poor in spirit, mourn, are meek, are persecuted, etc.'

At the end of each Beatitude there is a promise of what lies ahead for those on this particular path. Interestingly, the promise

for the first and last Beatitude is of *all of the kingdom – now*.
'Blessed are the poor in spirit, for theirs is the kingdom of heaven',
and 'Blessed are those who are persecuted for righteousness' sake;
for theirs is the kingdom of heaven'. For the other six, the promise
is a *part of the kingdom – in the future*. Those who mourn will be
comforted; those who are meek will inherit the earth; and so on.
This balance of 'all of it now' and 'parts of it later' expresses the
paradox in the teaching of Jesus that the kingdom has come
among us, and yet we are to pray for its coming. There is a both a
'now' and a 'not yet' aspect to the Christian faith.

A further symmetry, evident in the Beatitudes, is that the fourth
and the eighth are both about *righteousness*. One is about hungering for it, and the other about suffering persecution because of it.
Either way, maturity in God's sight is about a deep affinity with
the cause of righteousness as something we eagerly seek after, and
are also willing to suffer for. That suggests that the wimpish
nature of the Beatitudes cannot stand. Working and fighting for
righteousness does not fit with a weak approach to life. It certainly did not work out like that in the life of Jesus.

Their significance

Although the Beatitudes do seem to fulfil the same role as the Ten
Commandments in the Old Testament revelation, they are saying
something very different. Their style and thrust are so positive.
Beginning not with 'Thou shalt not ...', but rather 'You are blessed
...', they overflow with affirmation, accepting love, and reassurance. Here, clearly, we are in the realm of grace, rather than law.
Blessing, gift, hope, encouragement, grace; these are the foundations on which the kingdom announced by Jesus is built. That
speaks to the depths of who we are, for so often we are actually
more at home 'trying hard to be good', than we are in receiving

the goodness and gift of God's love. The Beatitudes take us into a whole new realm of living by and in the grace of God.

Their scope

We cannot limit the Beatitudes to the safety of the devotional life, or just our inner attitudes, though that is where they need to take root. They touch the whole of life. It is not just our relationship to God, or to our inner self, that is addressed; they speak rather to every aspect of living. They speak to our relationships with those who are closest to us, and to our work context (or lack of it). They also address the culture, values and political structure of the country in which we live. Our attitude to, and actions in connection with, the major issues in today's world, from environmental pollution to the deep-seated hostilities and injustices which so afflict our world, also come within the scope of the Beatitudes. All of life comes under the light of these remarkably few words.

The Beatitudes speak to the whole of life. We must allow them to address us that fully.

ON THE BEATITUDES
*The more we explore their implications
the more seems to remain unexplored.
Their wealth is inexhaustible.
We cannot plumb their depths.*

John Stott, *Christian counter-culture*

UNLOCKING THE BEATITUDES

Through the pages of history, and more widely in our 'Christian' culture, the Beatitudes have suffered serious misinterpretation. That may explain why they have fallen off the church's agenda. We have become confused by the interpretations placed on them. They seem to be so other-worldly and unattainable, and impossible to practise in 'real' life.

Some have sought to find a way out of this dilemma by thinking that they only apply to individuals in their own inner life. Some have suggested that they simply reflect different personality types; with the shrinking violets practising meekness, and the aggressive ones among us being those who suffer persecution – even if we have to admit it may be for their pigheadedness rather than 'for righteousness' sake'!

So how can we ever know what Jesus really meant by the Beatitudes? Fortunately the answer is rather obvious and accessible. We can know what they are about for one very clear reason. The Beatitudes are about the characteristics of the children of the kingdom, children of the heavenly Father. That being so, there is one supreme role model for such a calling, namely Jesus Christ himself.

How Jesus lived is the key to the interpretation of the beatitudes. He is the living embodiment of these truths. His whole life is therefore a commentary on them. Once we have this bedrock then we can draw on other material such as the rest of the Sermon on the Mount, the servant songs of Isaiah and the Psalms as great seams from which to mine further insights about the Beatitudes. All the time we will need to come back to the life, and teaching, of Jesus Christ, as the key to their interpretation.

OUR ROUTE THROUGH THE BEATITUDES

An explanation of the layout of this book is needed here.[1] The Beatitudes are grouped together in *pairs*. One reason for doing this is simply that they fit together like that. Indeed there is also a symmetry between the first four and the second four which is explored in the course of the book.

A further reason for this pairing is an important practical issue. If these truths are to be lived, and not just studied, we are most likely to do that if we can construct a simple rule of life, or *way of life* out of these sayings. Having four themes may well be helpful to that end.

This pairing is given further emphasis by there being a *reflective chapter* after each pair of Beatitudes. So there are four parts to the book, each including two chapters exploring two Beatitudes followed by a chapter considering how these truths might shape Christian living today.

As a further aid to engaging with the Beatitudes there is a *meditation* at the end of each chapter on a Beatitude. Where more than one reading, hymn or prayer is given,[2] it is intended that this will enable a different selection to be used where the meditation is used repeatedly. The meditations are suitable for individual or group use. Where they are used in a group, it is suggested that *reflections* be done in silence rather than as a discussion. The plural form (we/us) is used. This is done not only with groups in mind but also for individuals. The personal pronouns (I/me) can, of

---

1 All Bible references are from the *New Revised Standard Version*, unless otherwise stated.

2 All collects are from the New Lectionary of the Church of England, unless otherwise stated.

course, be substituted. However, individuals are encouraged to use the plural form as a reminder that even when we pray on our own, we are never alone in our praying. In prayer Christians join their prayers with the prayers of all God's people.[3]

A final chapter gives some concluding consideration to my primary hope in writing this book that it will lead not simply to a fresh understanding of the Beatitudes but to a *living expression* of this remarkable truth. That living expression needs to take place not only in and through the life of the church, but as individual Christians seek to give expression to their faith not least as a contribution to a culture in search of values rich enough to sustain its life.

May God give us His blessing to enable these truths to shine through the life and witness of the followers of Christ, whether as those gathered in the worshipping community, or as those scattered around the world in daily living.

3 Published at the same time is the final *Emmaus* initiation course workbook, *Your kingdom come*, which has a six-session study module on the Beatitudes.

PART ONE:
Open living

Being poor in spirit does not mean:

- it is holy to be poor – the Bible consistently sees it as an injustice and affliction and is never romantic about real poverty. Choosing poverty (or a simple lifestyle) is different
- it is holy to put yourself down – 'I'm useless ...', 'I'm no good ...', 'I'm a failure ...'. We say things like this to provoke people to say how wonderful we are. False humility is a form of pride. The person unable to love themselves cannot stop thinking about themselves
- it is good to grovel – God is angry when we abuse or 'put down' his creatures and creation. Jesus never behaved like a doormat. He knew how to stand his ground.

Rather it is about ...

- trusting God: not playing God in our own lives. Jesus prayed!
- acknowledging our needs. Jesus asked for water, company, etc.
- being interdependent, rather than independent – independence is a necessary (teenage) stage in life, but full humanity is found in being open to others, God and all creation.

ONE

SAYING YES TO LIFE

Blessed are the poor in spirit,
for theirs is the kingdom of heaven.

What a way to run a universe, start a new religion, and promote an alternative way of life for planet earth – to suggest that life is found in being poor. Today, of course, the image consultants and spin doctors would never allow it. 'First impressions', they would tell us, are all-important. As a lead focus and soundbite this will not do. You will attract the wrong sort of person, scare away the mass market, and confuse the rest. It just won't work.

Only it has! It has inspired some of the greatest manifestations of the human spirit, from Francis of Assisi to Mother Teresa. It has shaped whole communities, monastic and missionary, given hope to countless people who have found themselves at the bottom of life's pile, and guidance to some of the most influential people in history.

But it does puzzle. Not least is this so in the West and in developed countries where its message chips away at the very foundations of our culture and personal agendas. Its impact is most puzzling in the countries of Christendom where the proposition that God's blessing rests on the poor in spirit suffers from several handicaps. It clashes with the values of a consumer culture; runs counter to our perceptions – endlessly reinforced by the myths of advertising – that happiness lies in having much; and confuses us because we struggle to make sense of what Jesus meant.

MAKING SENSE OF POVERTY

There are two major obstacles that stand in the way of our hearing what this Beatitude is about. The first concerns what Jesus meant. Did he mean it is good to be poor? Or did he mean that an attitude of poverty is pleasing to God? Both lead to a dead end.

What we do know is that Jesus was well acquainted with the poor and with poverty. His own life was hardly a great materialistic success story. 'Borrowed' is written all over his life; from the borrowed stable in which he was born, the borrowed boat from which he preached, the borrowed houses he lived in while on his travels, the borrowed room in which he inaugurated the eucharist, to the borrowed grave in which he was buried. Not only that, but he was counted the friend of the poor. The ordinary people were the ones who flocked to hear him, the sick, lame and lepers cried out to him for healing. Those on the margins of society – prostitutes, publicans, tax collectors, foreigners and especially Romans – were the ones he was continually welcoming in to this 'kingdom' about which he preached.

Yet Jesus never glamorized poverty. He knew it too well to be romantic about it. He saw it, rather, as an evil to be eradicated, and preached against the hoarding of wealth. He saw the destructive impact in people's lives of the lack of necessities and of the consequent suffering of having to spend all your energies just to survive. The only poverty he commends is a freely chosen laying aside of what you have. The voluntary simplicity of lifestyle to which he called the disciples when they 'left their nets', and to which he challenged the rich young ruler in his command to 'forsake all and follow me', were characterized by a *freely chosen* way of life, not one imposed by a harsh and unjust political and economic order. We simply cannot reduce this Beatitude to a romantic celebration of poverty. Jesus was too aware of the way that lack of necessities was a deep affliction under which many people laboured.

The second way in which we struggle with this Beatitude is when we take it to mean a negative attitude to ourselves. How this text has often been interpreted stands as a major obstacle to our hearing it today. All too easily it is thought to be encouraging an attitude of self-rejection expressed in such terms as 'I'm useless', 'I'm no good', 'I'm stupid' and the many other negatives with which our inner dialogue so constantly afflicts us. Is this what Christianity is really all about – a great big inner put-down? It certainly does not square with Jesus' joyful acceptance of his own nature. He knew he was loved by God, that was his starting point. Uriah Heap is not a role model for the poor in spirit.

FOR CRYING OUT LOUD!

So what was it about the poor and about poverty that provoked Jesus Christ to begin the Sermon on the Mount with this striking commendation of the poor? Indeed what was it in the poor that drew Jesus to them throughout his ministry? What was this affinity which he had with the suffering, the oppressed, the rejected and the misfits?

The very fact that the poor were the ones who came to Christ gives us a clue. The scribes, Pharisees and rulers of the synagogues also came; but only to find some way of bringing Jesus down, looking for questions that would trick and trap him. All because they saw in Jesus a threat to their positions and plans.

The 'poor' came with a very different agenda. They were looking for answers, seeing in Jesus a source of hope and rescue. In the gospels they are the ones ready to ignore the established rules of social behaviour in their desperate search for answers to their deepest needs. The woman with the issue of blood pushes through the crowd to touch the hem of Jesus' garment. Zacchaeus ignores all thoughts of the sort of behaviour seemly for a bank manager and climbs a tree for a glimpse of Jesus – and what a view he gets! Bartimaeus shouts so loudly that people tell him not to disturb the place and cause a fuss, until Jesus calls him forward – then the same people are all over him! The poor are those desperate enough to ignore social rules and cry out for help. Crying out loud is what marks them out. They are the ones who are not content with the present set-up. They are looking for answers.

The life of Jesus resonates with the poor at a deeper level than their evident desire to hear what he had to say and receive what he had to give. They were on the same wavelength as him; journeying through life on the same path. That path was an attitude of openness to resources and help from beyond. It was a path which recognized that no one is complete in themselves, and that life is found by being open to God, life, others and all creation.

It is really only the poor in spirit who can, actually, have anything,
because they are the ones who know how to receive gifts.
For them everything is gift.
Simon Tugwell, *The Beatitudes*

TRACING LIFE TO ITS SOURCE

Here we touch the heart of this Beatitude. It was argued in the Introduction that the Beatitudes are in the first place a description of the life of Christ, the child of the kingdom. Then, by extension, they are also a description of any child of God; that is, of the life of all who choose to live within the magnetic field of that kingdom.

If that is so then we need to ask where we see Jesus Christ exhibiting true poverty of spirit. We certainly cannot trace any rejection of material things – he gained a reputation as a party-goer and as someone who enjoyed wine. We also see in him someone with a striking ability to enjoy everything without the need to own anything. We certainly cannot trace any sense of self-abnegation, wimpishness, or negative self-talk that so easily passes as 'humility' and poverty of spirit today. Rather we see something very different, namely a relaxed ability to affirm his own worth and value to God and his nature as reflecting something of the glory of God. Hence the series of great 'I am's' in John's gospel: 'I am the Bread of Life', 'I am the Light of the World', 'I am the Good Shepherd'.

One place where we meet this openness to others, and to God as The Other, is in Jesus' baptism. Though without sin, he freely chose to be open to all that God had in store for those who submitted themselves to John's baptism. As he emerged from the waters the heavens opened, the Spirit descended and Jesus heard words of deepest affirmation:

'You are my Son, whom I love; with you I am well pleased.'
(Luke 3:22)

Far from being 'poor in spirit' leading to putting oneself down, Jesus shows and experiences that it issues rather in a strong sense of self-acceptance as the result of experiencing divine acceptance. No wonder Jesus said that those who dare to be poor in spirit will find the kingdom of heaven opening up to them. He knew the truth from his own life. He discovered it in baptism, and many times thereafter.

The key characteristic of Jesus which emerges from the portrait of him in the gospels is that he is not someone self-contained, some perfect sealed-unit approach to humanity, but rather a person unusually open to life at every level. Open to God, able to hear his will ('man does not live by bread alone but by every word that proceeds from the mouth of God'), not some totally competent super-spiritual freak. Christ's attractive humanity stems from the same source, namely being open to God the Father as the One from whom he receives trustworthy definition of himself as chosen, loved and called into the will of God.

———————————

Self-rejection is the great enemy of the spiritual life
because it contradicts the sacred voice that calls us 'Beloved'.

Henri Nouwen, *Life of the Beloved*

———————————

FROM ANOTHER ANGLE

This picture of Jesus as the One open to life helps us to come at poverty of spirit from a different angle and so gain fresh glimpses of how it is to work out in our lives. Here are some of the ways that we can gain access to the riches of this Beatitude for our own lives.

Blessed are those who know their need of God; all life opens up before them. This catches something of the ability of Christ to be open to receive grace, vocation, wisdom not as his possession but as gift in the moment. It is this understanding that underlies the apostle Paul's teaching about the gifts of the Spirit. He does not see them as our possessions which once experienced we own in perpetuity, but as resources that come to us in the moment, as needed.

The person who is poor in spirit is thus open to receive strength and help, as well as wonder and joy, from whatever source it comes. Indeed such people see insight, strength and wisdom in the most unlikely sources. Mother Teresa called the dying poor her gems. It is this that opens up the kingdom of heaven to those who have chosen the Way of Christ.

Enjoying the give and take of life. Jesus takes this starting point in his teaching, of affirming the poor in spirit, in order to call us to a proper creaturely dependence. It is a message of particular relevance to our world where we have created a society which thinks that independence is the ultimate sign of mature humanity. The truth is that independence is actually the teenage stage in life, set between early dependence and the full humanity of *interdependence*. Poverty of spirit is about this capacity, or rather choice, to stay open to others and to life.

It may well be that one of the major problems within marriages is that people are seeking to become independent, rather than interdependent. There is a proper place for dependence in the marriage relationship as in all of life. This makes sense in view of the fact that our earliest relationships shape the rest of our patterns of relating. Being willing to receive help, be taught new things, be shown how to develop particular skills or handle situations better, is often a threatening thing to engage in. It requires true poverty of spirit; that is, a readiness to recognize the truth of what help we yet need and then to dare to seek that help.

A learning attitude to life. Scott Peck, in his bestselling book *The Road Less Travelled*, uses the illustration of map making. He points out how clever early maps were, yet to our eyes – with several centuries of map making behind us – they look laughably childish. The point that Scott Peck makes is that as we grow up all of us are continually revising our 'map of reality'. The problem is that too many of us settle, by our mid-twenties, with the map we have drawn by that stage in life. All additional information has to be squeezed into our existing plan, or else discarded. What we should be doing, if we wish to stay fully alive, is to keep reworking our map of reality as each new insight is gained. This is what it means to be poor in spirit. It is the opposite of a closed mind, of having life all sussed out and sewn up. To be open to life, to learning and to growing is what Jesus identifies as the first step into true humanity.

When we think we are absolutely right,
we stop seeking new information.
To be right is to be certain, and to be certain stops us from being curious.
Curiosity and wonder are at the heart of all learning.

John Bradshaw, *Healing the shame that binds you*

Refusing to settle for less. One of the striking features of the poor as portrayed in the ministry of Jesus, and in his teaching, is that they will not take 'no' for an answer. They know that life depends on it. So Bartimaeus does not mind who he embarrasses just as long as he can win the ear of Jesus. The parables of the persistent neighbour, and the poor widow who pestered a judge, show this same characteristic of the poor. For them, faith in Jesus decides matters of life and death. Being poor in spirit involves holding on to our vision of what could and should be, and refusing to be moved until we find the way through. It is this often earthy zeal for life that characterizes the poor, and establishes an affinity between them and Jesus. Our comfortable settling-for-less, and letting go of great dreams and visions, distances us from Him.

SAINTS ALIVE

Far from poverty of spirit being a cringing, weak and self-deprecating attitude to life, it is the source of true vitality and authentic holiness. The saints have always been those people who seem most fully alive. In popular culture they may appear 'other-worldly' in a negative sense – prim, proper, cold, closed, correct, without moods or passions. In fact, when you read their lives, they turn out to be the most human of people. They certainly have something of the child within them, able to wonder at the world, themselves and others; able to enjoy the present moment and able to have fun. They are the ones who live life to the full, because they are alive to life – that is to God, others and the whole of creation.

It is in that openness that God is encountered. Which is just what the Beatitude promises, that those who are poor in spirit will find the kingdom, or presence and action of God, opening up all around them, for faith is the bedrock on which the life of those who are poor in spirit is built. It is an open, trusting attitude, to life; but above all to God himself.

If we are radically poor before God, we are also radically gifted.
This is the other side of our creatureliness.

Luke Johnson, *Sharing possessions*

SIGNPOSTS ON THE WAY

The Beatitudes act like signposts on the road of life. When we face new, testing and hard choices, we do well to listen to these Beatitudes and to the direction in which they point us. They act often as a means of focusing God's vocation to us at particular junctures in life.

In my first book, *In the crucible*, I wrote about a time in the preaching ministry when, like the persistent neighbour, I knew that I had 'nothing to set before them'. That sense of lack, of poverty, led me into a sustained period of prayer out of which a fresh encounter with God as Spirit resulted. Acknowledging my poverty opened for me the windows of heaven.

We talk, rightly, about poets, artists, musicians and writers being 'inspired'. It is a way in which our culture, unconsciously, acknowledges the truth of this Beatitude – that creativity is a co-operative venture with that which is beyond us. Only by recognizing that we are in a partnership can any creative work proceed. The 'artist' is working with their material (whether music, clay or people, etc.), with their own inner abilities, and also – as the Christian sees it – in all these factors, and beyond them, with the creative Spirit of the living God.

This partnership with God, and with the whole of life, is what this first Beatitude calls us to enter so that we might find the fullness of life which God has planned for us.

Meditation

Blessed are the poor in spirit; for theirs is the kingdom of heaven.
We come before you as those created to enjoy your life and grace
We rejoice that you open your kingdom to all who seek your Way

READING

> *I sought the Lord, and he answered me;*
> *he delivered me from all my fears.*
> *Those who look to him are radiant;*
> *their faces are never covered with shame.*
> *This poor man called, and the Lord heard him;*
> *he saved him out of all his troubles.*

The angel of the Lord encamps around
*   those who fear him, and he delivers them.*
Taste and see that the Lord is good;
*   blessed is the man who takes refuge in him.*
Fear the Lord, you his saints,
*   for those who fear him lack nothing.*
The lions may grow weak and hungry,
*   but those who seek the Lord lack no good thing.*
  (Psalm 34:4–8)

HYMNS

Will you love the 'you' you hide
if I but call your name?
Will you quell the fear inside
and never be the same?
Will you use the faith you've found
to reshape the world around
through my sight and touch and sound
in you, and you in me?
John L. Bell and Graham Maule

O may this bounteous God
*   Through all our life be near us,*
With ever joyful heart,
*   and blessed peace to cheer us;*
And keep us in his grace,
*   and guide us when perplexed,*
And free us from all ills
*   In this world and the next.*
Martin Rinkart tr. Catherine Winkworth

REFLECTION

> *What are the riches and resources that sustain our life, and for*
>   *which we give thanks?*
> *What does our poverty prompt us to call out to God for?*
> *Where might God be calling us to bring a fresh openness to Him,*
>   *others, and life itself, or specific help from beyond the normal*
>   *horizon of our life?*

Blessed are the poor in spirit; for theirs is the kingdom of heaven.

PRAYERS

> *Almighty God,*
> *in Christ you make all things new;*
> *transform the poverty of our nature*
> *by the riches of your grace,*
> *and in the renewal of our lives*
> *make known your heavenly glory;*
> *through Jesus your Son our Lord,*
> *who is alive and reigns with you,*
> *in the unity of the Holy Spirit,*
> *one God, now and for ever. Amen*
> Collect for the 2nd Sunday after Epiphany

> *O God, forasmuch as without you*
> *we are not able to please you;*
> *mercifully grant that your Holy Spirit*
> *may in all things direct and rule our hearts;*
> *through Jesus Christ your Son our Lord,*
> *who is alive and reigns with you,*
> *in the unity of the Holy Spirit,*
> *one God, now and for ever. Amen*
> Collect for the 19th Sunday after Trinity

Mourning does not mean

◆ only, or even primarily, the grief we feel when someone we love dies
◆ being a killjoy – having a long-faced and judgemental attitude to life
◆ being a pessimist – Jesus overflowed with hope and true confidence in God.

Rather it is about ...

◆ grieving about the pain and injustice in the world
◆ feeling God's pain about how far things are from His purposes
◆ owning the fact that we are part of the problem
◆ refusing to run from pain – ours or others'.

———————————

TWO

MIND THE GAP

Blessed are those who mourn;
for they will be comforted.

An elderly woman turned up for the first time at a service in her parish church. She was met by the churchwarden who, doing a good job of welcoming newcomers, shook her by the hand. The moment he did so the woman burst into tears. All at once the church had two distressed people on their hands – the woman and the churchwarden. After helping her to a seat and fetching her a glass of water those around her asked what the matter was. Looking up at the church-warden she said, 'You are the first person to touch me for three years!' That seemingly minimal welcome had overwhelmed her.

A world away, young people are involved in development projects in the two-thirds world. One of the key figures in such projects told me that most people so engaged are motivated, not as is commonly supposed by love, but by anger. He was not saying this as a criticism but simply as an observation. He went on to say that their anger was about the injustice of the situation, which had provoked them to feel 'something should be done about that'. They then found themselves caught up in bringing about an answer to the prayer for justice implicit in such an attitude.

Two respected Christian men were both secret drinkers. Almost by chance they discovered each other's guilty secret. Realizing their lives were falling apart they agreed to help each other find a way out. It was a long and painful journey with plenty of downs as well as an eventual long-term journey out of that destructive addiction. How do we know about their story? They were the two men who founded Alcoholics Anonymous (AA), a movement and organization through which countless millions have found help, hope and strength to bring about change in their lives.

These three diverse stories have a common theme. They are about mourning.

Different though the setting was, in each situation there was an awareness of something wrong in life. With it came a willingness to face that truth and the strength to do something about it. Their very willingness opened a door of opportunity and gave them a key ability with which to unlock the situation; whether as initiator of change, or recipient of the change brought about by others. For the woman it was her own immediate world of personal loss – her husband had died three years before. For the young people it was the wrong they saw in the world around them. For the founders of AA, the wrong was at first simply in them, but became a wrong that others were experiencing and that they were then able to address.

GOOD MOURNING

In the ten steps of the AA recovery programme, committing oneself to this 'Higher Power', through which strength comes, follows on after the first step which well illustrates the true nature of mourning:

We admitted we were powerless over drink and that our lives had become unmanageable.

Hence the title for this chapter – 'Mind the Gap'. Comfort, meaning strength, is given to those who do mind about the gap. There is a necessary visionary element in true mourning. It is the fruit of seeing a distance between what is hoped for and what is currently experienced. For the Christian, the starting point in this mourning is personal confession and repentance. We dare to face and own our own wounds before attempting to help others, and take the beam out of our eye first before helping to remove the speck in the other person's eye.[1] So mourning is the capacity to face the gap between present reality and perceived good. It is lifting off of hope that has been ignited by the mixing of faith in God (poor in spirit) with acknowledged painful past experience (mourning).

Too easily this Beatitude has been taken to encourage a dour, long-faced and negative attitude to life. But that is not what Jesus is saying.

Another danger in trying to understand this Beatitude is that we fail to take the sheer courage and hard work of mourning seriously. It is important to note that Jesus said 'Blessed are those who mourn ...', rather than 'Blessed are those who are bereaved ...' We know with greater clarity today how mourning has various stages – of denial, anger, blaming, and integrating. All too easily this mourning is something which we run from. 'I will never trust them again ...' 'I've learned not to share my real feelings any more ...' 'That is the end of prayer/religion/hope as far as I am concerned ...' These are all expressions, understandable though they are, of retreat from mourning. Bereavement happens to us, mourning is a choice. A choice to turn and face the pain and work through it to a better and more whole future.

Jesus is commending and affirming those who have the courage to face and own their pain, to address it, without abandoning the

---

1 I have written more fully about this in the chapter entitled 'Good Grief', in my book on prayer, *An affair of the heart* (Highland, 1994, reprinted 1998).

hope which created the 'gap' in the first place. We see it demonstrated in his own life.

---

*Becoming comfortable with myself unmasked
is the first step in genuinely accepting others.*

Gerard Broccolo, *Vital spiritualities*

RUNNING FOR COVER

Repentance is a fundamental expression of the mourning Jesus is pointing us towards in this Beatitude. It is about facing the reality of our human predicament, and our own part in our particular problems. It is also about owning our part in the wider pain, injustice and suffering in today's world.

Sadly, when we begin to touch these raw nerves of our own frailty, we tend to run for cover, thereby cutting ourselves off from the grace that could be ours. We may, for example, have a personal preference for communicating what we think about situations, rather than what we feel; or the reverse. If we will not address that relative weakness, then we run for cover in the response with which we are more familiar. Or it may be a matter of preferring to be active rather than reflective in response to life. Both have a part to play, but always running into the response we feel most comfortable with is a failure to mourn, to face an imbalance in our own responses to life.

For some there is a real sense of sadness, loss of faith (in God or others) stemming from painful experiences in the past. Mourning is a willingness to face those painful feelings and find a way through. When we fail to do so they actually shape the whole of our living, for we spend our time hiding from what needs to be faced.

In Christ we see a different way. A way of facing, owning, working through the gaps that appear in life – and discovering there is life beyond them.

JESUS IN MOURNING

There are at least three accounts in the gospels of Jesus weeping; not that mourning is only found where weeping takes place. Jesus' whole ministry can be seen in the light of this Beatitude for it was his evident 'minding the gap', between what God desired and what life seemed to have 'on offer' for most people around him, that energized and gave focus to his mission. From this perspective, the great underlying theme of his ministry was his refusal to accept current experienced reality as God's will, or to sit down under what seemed like impossible odds to bring about change. These incidents of weeping are instructive in unpacking the meaning of this second Beatitude.

The first occasion is the most obvious and basic sense we associate with the idea of mourning, for it describes – in the shortest verse in the Bible – the response of Jesus to the death of Lazarus. We are simply told, 'Jesus wept.' Those two words speak volumes about the humanity of Jesus. He felt the way we do when someone we knew and loved has died. And this despite the context which makes it clear that Jesus knew he was on the way to raise Lazarus from the dead. Jesus' demonstration of resurrection, as in his own life, did not bypass the way of the cross; he experienced and faced the pain and grief of the situation. His tears were of sorrow for the whole family and community and for his own sense of loss and distance ('the gap') between him and Lazarus. The strength ('comfort') which Jesus experienced was first in discerning the will of the Father that he should stay away for several days, and subsequently in knowing that the Father intended to raise Lazarus from the dead. No doubt his enforced distance from his mourning friends, and the consequent stillness brought about by that waiting, played an important part in this discerning and strengthening process.

There have been a number of striking instances of this same process of grief leading to strengthening in service to others in recent years. Gordon Wilson, whose daughter was killed in the sectarian bombing of the Remembrance Day Service at Enniskillin in Northern Ireland, expressed forgiveness of the bombers and dedicated the rest of his life to the peace process in that land. He later became a senator in the Dublin parliament. The parents of Lisa Betts, a teenager who died as the result of taking the drug Ecstasy, have given themselves to a campaign to alert teenagers, and their parents, to the dangers of drug taking.

The second occasion when Jesus wept, was on his way to Jerusalem to confront the powers that be, in church and state, in that capital city. We read:

> As he came near and saw the city, he wept over it, saying, 'If you, even you, had only recognized on this day the things that make for peace! But now they are hidden from your eyes. Indeed, the days will come upon you, when your enemies will set up ramparts around you and surround you, and hem you in on every side. They will crush you to the ground, you and your children within you, and they will not leave within you one stone upon another; because you did not recognize the time of your visitation from God.' (Luke 19:41–44)

Here we see so clearly the gap between what Jesus longed to give – the good future which he knew the Father had in mind for the city – and current reality. It was this gulf that fuelled his grief. The pain of disappointed hopes, dashed possibilities and a longed-for opportunity to express love and compassion, was the source of Jesus' grief. No true mourning, in harmony with this Beatitude, is possible without an awareness of the hope that is being dashed by present events.

Yet it is in facing this pain and gulf that the comfort comes. Running from the pain distances us from the divine aid that would otherwise be God's gift to us. When we do turn away a double grief is experienced by God. There is both the grief of the original situation and then also the grief that results from our missing the invitation to be part of his redeeming response to that situation. How easily we choose that option by turning away from pain, in ourselves and in others – often simply by 'keeping busy', rather than daring to be still.

The third occasion on which Jesus was in evident distress was in the Garden of Gethsemane where we are told that his sweat was like drops of blood. Here Jesus is engaging at the deepest personal level with the ultimate gap between humanity and God which he had come to bridge. He here experiences that gap as a great impending gulf opening up before him, and from which he naturally shrinks – 'Father, if you are willing, remove this cup from me' (Luke 22:42). It is a reminder that this mourning, the ability to share with God in the pain of the gap between present experience and promised hope, is sometimes a costly calling. No wonder our culture shrinks from dwelling in its presence. Yet the Christian is one willing to hear that call and share in that creative pain.

Here again we see the fulfilment of the promise in this Beatitude, for 'an angel from heaven appeared to him and gave him strength' (Luke 22:43). Jesus discovers the dynamic of the second Beatitude at work in this moment of supreme testing. The assurance for us today is that where we have the courage to face the cause of our, and the world's, mourning we will also discover the strength to respond creatively and work to address the gap that has opened up before us.

A Christian is someone who shares the sufferings of God in the world.

Dietrich Bonhoeffer

LABOURING UNDER A
TRUE APPREHENSION

When archaeologists, around the turn of the next millennium, come to dig up the sites of late twentieth-century Western culture, the two artifacts they most need to discover in order to understand our society are the remote control unit and double glazing. They symbolize a community protecting itself from reality. The remote control speaks of our desire to be in control, with minimum personal inconvenience. Double glazing enables us to look out on the world, whilst minimizing its impact on us. The remote control and double glazing are great modern inventions. They are not the problem, but they do symbolize something in our culture which wants to maintain, or avoid noticing, the gap. In a multitude of ways we defend ourselves against the intrusion of the world around.

In this TV age where the troubles and suffering of the whole world are portrayed with amazing speed and clarity in our sitting rooms, it is easy to understand how we numb ourselves in the face of overwhelming problems and obstacles. Yet we have to find some way to be selective about these needs and resolve to participate in God's loving purposes in that situation; through prayer, interest, giving, working and supporting the work of others addressing such needs. We simply cannot claim to follow Christ and sit and watch, or just switch off, in face of the travails of this world; any more than we should try to play God in any or every such situation.

Yet there is another side, a different story. When historians come to write about the twentieth century, here in England, they will be able to point to a whole range of ventures where the followers of Christ have been at the forefront of dealing, as one writer put it, 'in the business of tears': Chad Varah's development of the Samaritans telephone work with the suicidal, Dame Cecily Saunders' pioneering work in the Hospice movement which has brought a new level of care for the terminally ill and their relatives, Relate and its work of counselling those seeking to sustain long-term relationships, and Cruse, serving the needs of the bereaved. These, and many other such ventures, are signs of this kingdom which dares to face the pain of human suffering. It really is a quite striking and extensive list that, rather like the missionary societies of previous centuries, indicates the healthy state of the Christian faith despite its perceived image.

Not that the story is confined to the work of the church. Amnesty International, Friends of the Earth, Greenpeace and many other groups, organizations and movements all illustrate this dynamic. In each there is a willingness to face, rather than run from, the pain, brokenness and injustice of the world. With that willingness to 'mind the gap' comes the discovery of the energy, will and ability to do something about the situation.

All of these ventures are labouring under a true apprehension of the situation, and taking their often costly and risky part in bringing about change.

ALLERGY TO REALITY

'Humankind', said T. S. Eliot, 'cannot bear very much reality.' Which is why, ever since the Garden of Eden in which the man and woman hid themselves, from God and from the consequences of their own actions, humanity has been on the run.

Nowhere is this more clearly demonstrated than in the growth of addictions. We not only recognize alcohol and drug addictions, but new terms like workaholics, shopaholics, even love-aholics (people addicted to the process of falling in love, but unable to sustain a committed relationship with another human being) draw our attention to the fact that ours is an addictive culture.

There is a right and healthy form of rest and recreation when we 'switch off'; but there is a difference between stopping and enjoying the world in which we live and the drivenness which hides either by 'numbing out', or through frantic (even 'frantic church') activity.

It is in the death of Christ that we find healing for this allergy to reality, life and God himself. All are addressed by that ultimate expression not only of God's minding the gap, but of his bridging the divide; namely the cross of Christ.

If we are to be fully alive and engage with reality, we have to find ways, opportunities and moments in which the pain within us and in the world around – seen as the tension created in any situation between what is and what could or should be – can be addressed. Without the willingness to face and address the pain there can be no gain. Cross-and-resurrection is the deepest theme of the universe itself. It is in aligning ourselves with that theme, as part of our baptismal identity, that we participate in life as God has intended and called us to experience it.

Resignation and denial are passive –
but sorrow is active, dynamic. It moves us on.
Kathy Galloway, *Struggles to love*

STRONG COMFORT

This is what the second Beatitude is about – an honest facing of the pain and brokenness in ourselves and others in such a way that energy is found to bring healing and help. The second part of the Beatitude helps unpack the first part. The promise is of comfort. Today we take that to mean a cup of tea and some reassuring words. Something like that was indeed involved in the first story, but comfort means something more robust – namely, strength. To comfort is to give strength to, to make strong; like 'proving' metal in such a way as to 'improve' it.

A well-known part of the Bayeux Tapestry has a picture of a group of people being prodded forward by a royal person who is using a 'goad' (a stick with a sharp point) into their backsides. Underneath are the words 'King William comforteth his troops'! No doubt they did not feel comfortable, but they certainly would have found new strength to keep going in the wake of such prodding. That is the meaning of the promise of comfort here, as it is also the meaning of the title 'Comforter', for the Holy Spirit. When Jesus called the Holy Spirit the 'Comforter' he was not speaking primarily in terms of soothing away our troubles, but rather of strengthening our wills to work to overcome the obstacles and testing that lie ahead of us.

This is a dominant aspect of the role of the Spirit as portrayed in the Old Testament, where the Spirit seems often to be 'the god of war'. What typically happened when the Spirit came upon people in those settings was that a crisis situation was addressed. The children of Israel had been in distress – provoked to mourn – and now strength was given to someone to be the means of mobilizing the whole community to participate in their own deliverance. Samson and Gideon were two such people who were equipped, in very different ways, to be part of God's rescue of the whole nation. Supremely one sees this in Moses through whom the whole nation was mobilized first to want, and then to be willing to work for, deliverance from Egypt. In their grief God's Spirit came to strengthen all through strengthening one. The book of Judges is the story of a long line of such strengthening acts of the Holy Spirit.

In each of the opening stories of this chapter, such strengthening is evident. The elderly woman was strengthened through the very gentleness of the welcome she received. The young people were strengthened by the anger within, and the founders of Alcoholics Anonymous discovered strength in each other and through their faith in God – what they were later to call their 'Higher Power'.

The promise of this Beatitude is that strength will be discovered wherever, at the personal or corporate level, we dare to trust God enough to face the brokenness of human existence, and to work through to a place where we find the strength to bring good out of failure.

Meditation

Blessed are those who mourn; for they will be comforted.
We come before you as those who know the brokenness of your world
We rejoice that you give us strength to share in your healing work

READING
> *I waited patiently for the Lord;*
> > *he turned to me and heard my cry.*
> *He lifted me out of the slimy pit,*
> > *out of the mud and mire;*
> *he set my feet on a rock*
> > *and gave me a firm place to stand*
> *He put a new song in my mouth,.*
> > *a hymn of praise to our God.*

Many will see and fear
    and put their trust in the Lord.
Blessed is the man who makes the Lord his trust.
(Psalm 40:1–4a)

HYMNS
    Where is thy reign of peace
        And purity and love?
    When shall all hatred cease,
        As in the realms above?

    When comes the promised time
        That war shall be no more,
    And lust, oppression, crime,
        Shall flee thy face before?
    L. Hensley

    Look around you, can you see?
    times are troubled, people grieve.
    See the violence, feel the hardness;
    all my people, weep with me.

    Walk among them, I'll go with you
    Reach out to them, with my hands.
    Suffer with me, and together
    We will serve them, help them stand.
    Jodi Page Clark

REFLECTION

> *Where are we most conscious of the gap between God's loving*
> *purpose and present reality?*
>
> *a. in our own lives,   b. in the world around us*
>
> *What strengthening do we desire from God to respond to those*
> *situations?*

Blessed are those who mourn; for they will be comforted.

PRAYERS

> *O God,*
> *who knowest us to be set in the midst*
> *of so many and great dangers, that by reason*
> *of the frailty of our nature we cannot always*
> *stand upright: grant to us such strength and*
> *protection, as may support us in all dangers,*
> *and carry us through all temptations;*
> *through Jesus Christ our Lord. Amen*
> Collect for the 4th Sunday after Epiphany (BCP)

> *Grant, we beseech you, merciful Lord,*
> *to your faithful people pardon and peace,*
> *that they may be cleansed from all their sins*
> *and serve you with a quiet mind;*
> *through Jesus Christ your Son our Lord,*
> *who is alive and reigns with you,*
> *in the unity of the Holy Spirit,*
> *one God now and for ever. Amen*
> Collect for the 21st Sunday after Trinity

THREE

OPEN LIVING

Blessed are your eyes, for they see,
and your ears for they hear.
Matthew 13:16

A businessman friend, who travels around the whole globe, recently told me a story about the disorientation he experiences as the result of so much travelling. He had flown out on a business trip, booked into the hotel and retired to bed. Around three o'clock in the morning the receptionist rang his room, apologized for disturbing him, told him there was an urgent telephone call and asked if he would take it. 'Yes,' he said, 'on one condition – that you tell me where on earth I am!' Waking up in the middle of the night he could not remember, quite literally, 'where in the world' he was.

Many of us feel like that, even without travelling much. We feel less and less sure we know 'where in the world' we are – or rather, what sort of world we are in. The familiar landmarks have gone and we easily feel disorientated.

There is a positive side to all this. We enjoy and value the freedom of our choice culture. But there is a price to pay. It is paid for in a loss of security and belonging; and in the loss of familiar patterns and places, rhythms and routines. The irony is that although we can go anywhere and 'do our own thing', we have problems finding our way. Life can sometimes seem like a desert – one vast trackless area. When 'anything goes' which way should we turn?

A COMPASS TO STEER BY

Many events in recent years have underlined the paradox in Western culture that whilst people seem resistant to, and distanced from, organized religion, they are nevertheless searching for meaning and a spiritual dimension to life. In this culture where 'anything goes' there is a desire to find the right way to go – to discover values by which to live.

The Beatitudes provide us with just that. Indeed they act like a compass by which we can find our way in a constantly changing culture with few clear landmarks or accepted values. This is particularly so when we approach the Beatitudes as four pairs, rather than eight individual sayings. Those four pairs can stand like the four points of a compass. They do seem to fit around four distinct themes. Seeing them as pairs helps to uncover otherwise hidden depths to these eight sayings of Jesus.

OPEN TO GOD

The first two Beatitudes (the poor in spirit, and those who mourn) suggest that being open to God is the first point on the compass.

We have seen how the poor in spirit are those who are open to life, able to receive it as gift, and ready to look for and find strength, wisdom and support, outside of and beyond themselves. It is the rich who are sent empty away. The hungry are the ones who are filled with good things, because they are the ones whose hands, hearts and whole lives are open to what lies beyond them.

The second Beatitude, about those who mourn, takes us further on into openness to the pain and limitations both of ourselves and of others around us. Once we dare to be receptive to the world around us – God, others and all creation – we discover that pain lies that way. We have all known something of what it means to be 'disappointed in love', whether the love was of another human being or some hoped-for, or worked-for, goal or prize.

Paul speaks of faith, hope and love as the primary virtues of the Christian faith. But faith – whether trusting God, others or the bridge across the river – does not always seem to 'hold'. Love can disappoint, and hope can die. Exercising faith, hope or love involves taking risks. Rather than deny this and tell us that 'it will all work out in the end', Jesus commends those who are willing to face the cost, the risk, and pain. The promise for them is that they will be strengthened. So mourning is another form of openness: openness to the pain of the world.

Jesus gave assurances that people who love life
and let go their hold on all that defends them
from the risks of love will not be lost.

J. Neville Ward, *Five for sorrow, ten for joy*

OPEN TO LIFE

In an important sense it can be said that the theme of these two Beatitudes is not simply openness to God, but being open to the whole of life. The poor in spirit are those who look beyond themselves and are receptive to the goodness of life. Jesus enjoyed other people's company, good food and wine, the beauty of creation, and the way they spoke to him of his Father. He was also deeply aware of the pain in the world and spent much of his short ministry addressing the multitude of human needs around him; and he sought to confront the roots of so much human misery stemming from unjust structures of social, political and religious life.

Certainly, we must not take 'open to God' in a narrowly religious or spiritual sense. Rather, what we see in Jesus is an openness to God in the whole of life. This included a willingness and ability to receive as well as give. As a twelve-year-old he is found in the Temple 'sitting among the teachers, listening and asking them questions'. He borrows Peter's boat, asks the woman at the well for a drink (surely because he was thirsty not as 'a good evangelistic ploy'), and pleads with his disciples for their company and support in Gethsemane. He was good at receiving.

Living by these first two Beatitudes today calls us to the same ability to learn and receive. Not least is this so because we live in a remarkably 'open culture'. There is a significant degree of honesty about emotions, a desire to 'get real' and a real passion (especially in many young people) about the injustices in the world, the needs of the poor and the sufferings of the environment. In many of our churches we need the openness and honesty in the culture around us to invade our 'niceness' with the breath of honesty and reality.

However, this raises an important issue that we need to address before considering further what being open to God, and the whole of life, might involve for the followers of Christ today.

NATURAL OR SUPERNATURAL?

Not all the illustrations used in the previous two chapters were necessarily Christian in origin. That raises an important question about the relationship between the Beatitudes and moral values in our society. Do the Beatitudes express values for all, or are they specifically and exclusively Christian? Are they natural to all people or something only made possible by faith encounter with Christ? The answer leads us to one of the many paradoxes of the Christian faith.

In one sense the Beatitudes are specifically Christian. They point to a conscious faith relationship between the disciple of Christ and the Father to whom he pointed. They are a description of the characteristics of those into whose lives God has broken – with his blessing. The very blessing in which they are all set is about communication between two parties – God and the follower of Christ. They are a description of the character of those who have entered the kingdom of God. Moreover, the Beatitudes, as we have already noted, cut across the norms and values of all cultures. Affirming mourning, meekness and mercy is 'counter-culture'. Here are the values of the kingdom, the new age inaugurated by Christ. As such they are 'upside-down values'; though properly understood they are 'upside-up' values, putting life back onto the basis it was designed to work on. Which leads us straight into the other side of this paradox.

In so far as the Beatitudes are putting things back 'the right way up', they are about the recovery of what has been lost; namely our humanity. In this sense the Beatitudes are profoundly natural, and are found – at least in some measure – 'occurring in nature'. Being poor in spirit is seen in all those who are only too aware of their own limitations of wisdom, skill, patience, ability, etc. The natural tendency is to deny, mask or run from this truth, but we all know it. The Beatitudes call us to face it. Equally, we see meekness in many scientists who are reduced to a sense of wonder and humility, as they explore the depths of the DNA code or the nature of black holes. Or consider the matter of mercy. The response to the work of Mother Teresa with the destitute of Calcutta, or the work of Diana, Princess of Wales, in caring for AIDS sufferers and for the victims of land mines, resonates strongly with people of all faiths and none. Yes, some would question what is achieved, or even the motives, but the actions are recognized as genuinely 'good'. There is a seam of mercy deep in the human heart. Consider the way in which, when death confronts people, one of the most urgent things they want to do is get in touch with friends and relatives from whom they have become alienated. There is a deep instinct for peace-making in the human heart – when it finds a chance to be expressed. Moreover, when we consider the ultimate motivation for all human behaviour we know that it is about the search for happiness. And what is the 'blessed' state into which these Beatitudes call us, other than that of finding happiness through experiencing God's blessing on our lives?

Every good man or woman is like Christ.
What else could they be like?

C. S. Lewis, *Prayer: Letters to Malcolm*

The work of the gospel, and of the Beatitudes in particular, is to mine these seams of rich humanity and bring them to the surface. All too often, cultures suppress and belittle these things. We need therefore to hold together both truths, namely that the Beatitudes are the 'most natural and human values in the world', and yet they are 'the truly supernatural gifting' that God gives to all who call on the name of Christ. At one and the same time we can expect to see at least echoes of them in all humanity; yet we need to look to God's revelation in Christ if they are to come to fullest expression in our lives.

LIVING IT OUT

We turn now to identify some of the implications for life today of this trusting openness to God, to which the first pair of Beatitudes call us. Bearing in mind the way in which the culture in which we live can be described as 'open to life', albeit with plenty of down-sides and blind spots, we need to consider what is distinctive about how these Beatitudes call us to be open to God in the whole of life.

Being good receivers. To be open to all that God gives us in life means learning to be on the receiving end of what he desires to give. Otherwise we will not be able to experience the blessing intended. This certainly involves us in prayer and the other means of grace. The hands of the believer open to receive the sacrament of communion well illustrate what it means to be poor in spirit. They are also a picture of the consequences of such poverty – access to God's life within our own lives. Here it is important to remember that it is not so much the doing of these actions (of prayer, communion, etc.) as the attitude of openness in which we come to them. Being open to receive is what opens the door to God's gifts.

That grace of God is not confined simply to 'spiritual' or 'religious' things. God gives to us in the whole of life, and often through other human beings. Martin Luther encouraged clergy to spend time with little children and with animals and 'all things that takes life blithely'. God speaks to us in the whole life. Every experience has the potential to be an expression of His communication with us – a kind of annunciation.

Furthermore, our calling is not just to be good receivers ourselves, but rather also to help those groups, organizations and systems which we are part of, to be good at receiving. Helping our families, churches and places of work to be good learners and receivers is part of the outworking of this principle of being open to God in all of life.

God reveals himself to the humble in the humblest things,
while the great who never penetrate beneath the surface
do not discover him even in great events.

Jean-Pierre de Caussade, *Self-abandonment to divine providence*

Making the right connections. Today's world is characterized by remarkable communications. We can 'speak' to someone on the other side of the globe by telephone or through the Internet. We can watch events thousands, and tens of thousands of miles away – at the very time they are taking place. We can consume fruits from all over the world so that there is hardly a 'season' for anything. However, all this communication is at the material and 'horizontal' level. What our culture is not so good at is making connections at the deeper level. Many of us relate to more people, at less depth, than our grandparents. More than that, the contemporary interest in spirituality indicates that we have starved ourselves of the deeper significance of our experiences of life. There is a hunger abroad for answers to questions of meaning and the purpose of our existence on this planet.

It is here that the life of Jesus is such a contrast to today's world. He lived, by modern standards, such a 'restricted' life, probably never travelling more than one hundred miles from his home town. He never moved beyond that provincial backwater of the Roman Empire. Yet he had such a rich awareness of life. He had learned to be open to life and to God to such an extent that he could see the hand of God, and hear the word of God, in a housewife losing a coin, a farmer sowing seed, lilies growing wild and a thousand other everyday events. He could also read human motives, discern 'the question behind the question' and see what could be, not just what was. He was seeing the deeper truths, making the right connections, and being alive to God and the fundamental issues of life. The Beatitudes call us to the same task in our day. That will involve us, among other things, in being good listeners – to God, life and other people.

Appreciation. That does not sound like a very dramatic and 'prophetic' action. It may make us feel like Naaman the leper who came to Elisha to be healed and was told to go and bathe seven times in the river. He was hoping for something more spectacular. We live in quite a 'hard-nosed' and 'hard-bitten' culture in which expressing appreciation is rarely considered important enough to be worth paying attention to. It is about giving expression to positive responses to situations and people.

In daily conversation it seems acceptable to complain about the government, the boss, the church, the media etc.; yet we are easily embarrassed if we attempt to express appreciation for any of these. Appreciation suggests we are naive, gullible, and do not realize that 'they are only in it for the money'. But to appreciate creation, the company of others, the benefits of modern technology, the uniqueness and vitality of others, is to be open to receive blessing through them. It is not for nothing that the eucharist – meaning 'thanksgiving' – is the central act of worship of the Christian church. Living in openness to life calls us to dare to affirm the many good and positive things in the world, and the work of others, around us. It is a call to live in thanksgiving.

I have had the privilege of working in places where one or two people have been consistently appreciative. It has lifted the spirits of all involved in the operation, made the hard work all seem worth while. They also, incidentally, were the people who gained the readiest hearing when they had a criticism to make, just because it was not their normal mode of speaking.

Stillness. It is difficult to find anything to express appreciation for if we never stop running through life. Certainly Jesus had a very pressured ministry, besieged by the sick, by those out to trick and trap him, and often frustrated by the blindness of his closest followers. But he made time to be alone, to stop, to reflect on life and to bring all his experience of life to God in prayer.

Our culture seems afraid of silence. We are regularly injected with music to lull us, not to sleep in our mother's arms, but to buy much in the aisles of the supermarket. We seem allergic to stopping and consequently shallow in many of our relationships. It may be that the popularity of traditional Gregorian chant in the musical charts reflects a desire to still the turmoil within. How interesting that this church music, with its simple rhythms which still the heart, is the one form of religious music that is connecting with today's world.

Both the Beatitudes concerning the poor in spirit, and the mourning, are invitations to stop and get in touch with what is happening around us, with our own responses and with the choices that are pleasing to God in the circumstances we face. Even in our churches we are too easily caught up with the rush and pressure of life. Certainly our worship needs to recover this creative stillness.

Our fragmented society needs a whole series of 'reflective pools',
places where the very deepest issues of life and death may be explored
and understood away from the cut and thrust of the market place.

Terry Waite, *Taken on trust*

Celebration. Stillness is not the only form of stopping. There is a place for its opposite, namely the processions into the Temple described in the Psalms. Life gives us plenty of cause for those communal acts of enjoyment. Indeed our culture still looks to the church to be the place that helps it with 'rituals that relate' at the key moments of life such as birth, marriage and death.

But there are other celebrations (both of joy and of grief) which may well be a particular way in which the church is called to serve the community. Certainly it is not all about events and services. Celebration is more about an attitude to life; an ability simply to stop and enjoy what is, rather than rush on to the next thing or try to squeeze one more achievement into an already packed schedule. Here appreciation, speaking out our gratitude for life and our awareness of the good things around us, can develop a spirit of celebration within, without any organized activity being needed.

Lamentation. This is the other side of celebration. It is the willingness to face the pain and tragedy that continually cross our journey through life. Here again, the Christian church has often served the wider community well in giving expression to these corporate moments of grief. The funeral of Diana, Princess of Wales, was simply the most visible of these. But other examples abound. One church held a memorial service to mark the tenth anniversary of the closure of the local pit, in order to allow the 'frozen anger' in the community to be given expression. Another had a special prayer vigil when a child was killed by a car while playing in the street. One church held a memorial service when a local hotel had to be demolished, since the church knew that many people in the community had strong associations with the place because their eighteenth or twenty-first birthday parties, wedding receptions and funeral wakes had been held there. Serving the community through such events is part of being open to life.

There is a hidden part of lamentation too, namely confession. As a culture we are very quick and ready to take others to court to compensate for misjudgements and things we have suffered at their hands. We are much slower to face our own responsibilities for the tragedies and disappointments of life. Repentance, though hard work, is also good and healthy work. The image of washing is often used as a picture of repentance. Like a good bath or shower, true owning up to the gap in our own lives between professed faith and preferred options can cleanse, revive and refresh us. It is a secret work, but with a very evident public face. 'Sorry' can be a most powerful word to speak in many of the most fraught situations in life.

SABBATH

One theme in scripture encapsulating so much of this openness to God in the midst of life is that of sabbath.

The kingdom of God, as we shall see in later chapters, is not only the focus of the Lord's Prayer and central to the teaching of Jesus, it also lies at the heart of the Beatitudes. But where did Jesus get this idea of the kingdom from? At one level it is hardly central in the Old Testament, except in the geographical and political sense of the kingdom under David and Solomon. But Jesus went out of his way to say that the kingdom of God is not like that. He was not in pursuit of political power. So where did the kingdom come from? One major root is this Old Testament theme of sabbath.

Beginning in Genesis the subject continues to reverberate throughout the Jewish scriptures. It is first introduced as an act of God. God celebrates sabbath. Whilst creation is done simply by a word, 'then God said', when it came to sabbath, God enters into his creation in order to enjoy it.

In a culture that has abolished Sunday as the traditional day of rest, the task of the church is to help in recovering, and finding fresh ways of expressing, this lost art of stopping, resting and enjoying what is.

Certainly in the scriptures, it is related to one day and expressed in the rhythms and routines of life. In our 'anything goes' culture, we can now do anything almost any time. It is a convenience culture. Yet have we not lost something by breaking up long-established patterns and rhythms in life? We cannot, and should not, attempt to put the clock back. Many Sunday trading laws (that allowed you to buy chicken and chips but not fish and chips, pornography but not a Bible) certainly needed removing. Moreover, we are living in a mobile and fragmented world. Somehow, however, we need to recover sabbath, doubtless in new ways that will surprise us and yet ring true with the past. It is an important part of the church's service of the wider community.

That recovery needs to be not simply in the church but for the world, developing ways of establishing sabbath – moments, routines, of stopping, appreciating, stillness, celebration and proper grieving, that can be energizing for the whole community.

If we are to develop and express lifestyles that are truly open to God and to the whole of life, we will need the gift and ordering of life that sabbath brings. It is a theme that enables us to express our commitment to live by the truths of these first two Beatitudes.

PART TWO:
Purposeful living

Meekness does not mean

◆ being weak and wimpish
◆ letting people walk over us: always giving in to others
◆ never disagreeing with anyone.

Rather it is about ...

◆ trusting God's help: they inherit (not 'own') the earth, receiving life as a gift from God rather than a possession to get and defend. The meek can enjoy the whole of life
◆ not grasping but trusting – waiting for God's moment and God's plans
◆ exercising life-giving authority (like Moses and Jesus) not domineering control, but devoting ourselves to God's agenda and priorities and trusting God with our needs.

FOUR

STRENGTH IN MEEKNESS

Blessed are the meek,
for they will inherit the earth.

Of all the Beatitudes there can be little doubt that this is the one with the worst press. In popular perception, meekness is weakness. So this Beatitude looks like a doormat ethic – an invitation to other people to walk all over us. Add to that the fact that the promise here is that the meek will inherit the earth, and the idea that this, of all Beatitudes, is the most unrealistic and idealistic, seems to have something going for it.

But does it? The two people in scripture described as meek are Moses and Jesus. Both confronted powerful and despotic rulers and one lost his life in doing so. That hardly fits with ideas of weakness. Yet Moses and Jesus did actually 'inherit' quite a bit of planet Earth. Moses led the children of Israel out of slavery to the Promised Land. Several thousand years later, and after many twists, turns and conflicts, the nation still does inherit that piece of land. Jesus, crucified as a disgraced criminal 'outside the city wall', has something like one third of the globe owning allegiance to him in some form. The the millennium celebrations indicate just what an influence he has had on human history; and how much he has inherited.

So maybe there is something in the Beatitude that connects more with the real world than might at first be thought.

ON BEING 'MEEKED'

If meekness does not mean weakness, then just what does it mean? An equestrian use of the word can help here. The term is used in the training of the Lipizzaner stallions from the famous Spanish riding school in Vienna. Before they can be trained to perform some amazingly complicated movements they have to be broken in. The term used is 'meeked'. It means to make biddable and responsive to the trainer.

That training is done because there is a very focused and specific outcome in mind. We see such a principle in every discipline of life. From football players to concert pianists and from able professors to skilled punters (of either kind!) the same process is at work. It begins with a clear goal and very specific focus. The one hundred metre runner, Linford Christie, was someone who perfected this sense of focus, not least at the start of each race. It is this choice that enables these people to submit themselves to intense discipline and costly sacrifices in order to achieve their goal. Winning a gold medal no doubt feels rather like inheriting the earth.

So meekness is about yielding to a clear goal and making the sacrifices to bring that about. This is something our culture is quiet about, for the goal seems rather to be that of keeping your options open, avoiding being trapped in any commitments, so that you can 'hang loose' and 'go with the flow'. Yet the people whom our culture admires, whether athletes, entertainers, business tycoons or icons of the young, are all people who have exercised considerable discipline to achieve their goals, whatever we might feel about the worth, or otherwise, of those goals. They have freely chosen to yield themselves to a 'higher agenda'.

Meekness is a real preference for God's will.
A. T. Pierson, *George Müller of Bristol*

THE HIGHER AGENDA

Meekness is another aspect of being poor in spirit. Both call us to live by drawing on resources from beyond ourselves. While the focus of the first Beatitude is on living in openness to all that God, life, creation and other people can give us (and call out of us), the emphasis in this Beatitude is not so much about resources for living as about our agenda in life. It is about discerning and following vocation. That word has become unduly restricted by being applied simply to work, and then only to a few roles in society – such as doctors, teachers, nurses and clergy. But vocation is about living the whole of life in response to a sense of call and purpose.

We see this wonderfully demonstrated in the life of Moses and especially in his call at the burning bush. His life story was all about burning. It began with burning anger as he saw the suffering of the children of Israel. Then, out of a sense of righteous indignation, he took the law into his own hands and killed the Egyptian who was harassing one of his own countrymen. It did not solve the problem. Rather, it created another, namely loss of respect and confidence from his own nation. 'Who made you a judge and a ruler over us?' The only solution was to get out. Far away, to what the Authorized Version calls 'the backside of the desert'; and for a long time – forty years.

During that wilderness and waiting period Moses' sense of justice continued to burn. It was in settling another dispute (this time without resorting to violence) that he met his wife. Forty years had not dampened the fires within him.

Then he stumbled across a burning bush. We will never know why God chose to reveal himself that way, but it could just have been because Moses, who knew all about fire that consumes – whether the physical sort that warms and cooks, or the moral sort that burns with indignation – would be likely to take another look if he saw a fire that could *burn yet not consume*. No wonder he took a second look.

But we need to take a second look too, for we miss the real miracle if we look only at the burning bush. *It was what took place inside Moses which was the real transformation* that has profoundly affected the world we now live in. The real miracle was on the inside; a changed heart. It happened in several stages.

First came a call to yield to a higher power, a greater Being than himself; hence the command to take off his shoes. It symbolized the presence of One for whom Moses should have respect, and led him to listen to and to obey this Other.

Then came a remarkable self-disclosure from God, in which he revealed that what had been on Moses' heart for four decades, had been on God's heart too – and for longer.

> Then the Lord said, 'I have observed the misery of my people who are in Egypt; have heard them crying on account of their task masters. Indeed, I know their sufferings, and I have come down to deliver them ...' (Exodus 3:7–8)

The third stage was something of a heart transplant. Here, in these words from God, was the same deep desire for justice, but it was touched by something lacking in Moses' burning passion, namely compassion. It is that compassion which touches and enters his heart and shapes the man in his new mission. He has been 'meeked': yielding to God's agenda.

Meekness means committing our lives to fulfil God's plans.
Michael Crosby, *Spirituality of the Beatitudes*

SPIRITUAL ENERGY

That experience began the process of strengthening Moses for the testing task which lay ahead. Far from his meekness – in saying yes to God's compassion and purposes – making him weak, it was the way in which he discovered strength.

The picture that comes to mind is of the hydro-electric plant. Before the dam is built or the turbines installed, the water flows downhill into the main stream and on out to the sea. Building the dam channels the flow. Now the waters are held back, later to be released with enormous, controlled power to drive the turbines that generate electricity. Here is vast power, harnessed to a higher purpose to serve the needs of many. It has been meeked.

Such an understanding of our engagement with the transcendent, namely that we find strength and true spirituality as we give ourselves to a higher agenda, contrasts sharply with much contemporary spirituality. The latter is usually seen as something 'marketed' to help us achieve a 'fuller life'. Biblical spirituality does actually bring that about, but through the step of faith by which we seek to discover and give ourselves over to God's purposes. This is expressed in the Lord's Prayer in terms of praying for the coming of God's kingdom and the doing of his will, both in our world (the big picture) and in our lives (the personal focus). That prayer is conspicuous in putting God's purposes ('your name, your kingdom, your will') ahead of our needs ('give us, forgive us, deliver us').

WHOSE SERVANT?

One particular incident in the life of Christ uncovers some striking truths about the nature of meekness. It is the well-known story of the foot washing, in the context of the Last Supper, on the eve of his crucifixion.

The first thing which emerges is that meekness is not about being pushed around by others, but rather about the strength that comes to a person when they are serving God's purposes. Peter was all for changing the rules of engagement, first saying he should be washing Jesus' feet and then, when Jesus insisted on doing it this way round, demanding a bath instead. On both occasions Jesus was making it clear that what Peter wanted was not on offer: it was foot washing or nothing. This toughness arose out of the awareness of Jesus that he was called to be the servant *of* God and a servant *to* the disciples. His ultimate calling was to do the will of the Father; not his own will, nor that of the disciples. How easily we confuse servant *to* with servant *of*. Our calling is not to fit in with everybody else's wishes, but rather to discern and do the will of God. This is the way of meekness.

The second thing is actually the prior point. It is about the inner security out of which Jesus initiated this remarkable servant act. The text reveals an inner self-acceptance and security that was the basis of the whole event.

> Jesus knowing that the Father had given all things in his hands, and that he had come from God and was going to God, got up from the table, took off his outer robe, and tied a towel around himself. Then he ... began to wash his disciples' feet. (John 13:3–4)

Clearly, meekness is not about being pushed around but about the strength to discern and choose the best option, and the inner security to do so. It is this that enables a person to be an agent of change. Self-acceptance and an inner sense of security are needed if we are to be agents of change in the world around us.

The key to the ability to change is a changeless sense of who you are, what you are about and what you value.

Stephen Covey, *The seven habits of highly effective people*

GOD OF THE GAPS

Meekness is strongly linked to the mourning of the previous Beatitude. Both depend on seeing another future, another way, another option, another agenda and having the courage to work to that end. Both are required if we are to bring into being that which at present does not exist. Both Beatitudes are built on hope, on the vision of a different outcome. With mourning it is about the courage to see the gap between what is and what could be; with meekness there then comes the courage to discern God's way, to address the gap and to look for divine strength to bring that future hope, at least in some measure, into reality.

However, seeing the gap between present reality and future possibility will often make us out of step with the world around us, and a puzzle to friends and enemies alike. Facing that gap may well get us into trouble before we see any hopes made reality.

In recent years two people, amongst many men and women, have been an inspiration and agents of profound change in the communities they serve. They have modelled meekness in the tough world of politics.

One such person is Vaclav Havel of the Czech Republic. In the former communist state of Czechoslovakia he was a poet and playwright, hardly a position that would seem to threaten the stability of the political structures. But he had a vision of a different and better country. It was of a country not only liberated from the *oppressive* 'lie' of totalitarian control but also of one not trapped by the *seductive* 'lie' of materialistic capitalism. It was the vision of a land where people were truly free and able to shake themselves free of the lies which distort so much of human life. He was a man with a grasp upon, or rather grasped by, reality – by a higher agenda.

With this vision burning within him, he began to write poetry. Amazingly he was put in prison for writing poems. As such he was not the first poet whom the state recognized as a threat to its power, for poets provoke people to think and to envisage a different future. Once people have a vision they are less likely to be satisfied with what is, and more willing to make the sacrifices to bring about the fulfilment of that vision. It was for the same reason that writers like Solzhenitsyn were imprisoned in the USSR.

Vaclav Havel must have had little hope or expectation of his ideas winning the argument or bringing down the state apparatus, but he kept on speaking about this other way of seeing life. Who could have imagined the turn of events that would result in his being, for a number of years, the president of his country? More than that, because of his poems, his plays and his work in the dissident group Charter '77, his was the crucial voice and mind that was the hinge on which many communist countries around Czechoslovakia swung in the heady days of the late 1980s and early 1990s. He has, in a real sense, inherited a large chunk of the earth.

The other person is Nelson Mandela. He too was fired by a vision. Raised in a royal household his early life seems to have many parallels with that of Moses. While Moses suffered exile for forty years, Nelson Mandela was exiled for a mere twenty-eight years – though without the freedoms that Moses experienced it doubtless would have seemed much longer. The powers that imprisoned him could certainly have expected that after so long an imprisonment the fire within him would have died down. But it did not. In fact it was purified. Gone was the commitment to violence and in its place a way of majestic reconciliation. The higher agenda of blacks and whites living as one community emerged deep within his soul.

The theme of a 'rainbow people', wherever it came from, spoke with the eloquent simplicity that only inspiration can bring into being. Staying with the colour imagery which had so torn apart and afflicted that nation over many decades, it yet – in just two words – put the nation's perception of race into a radically different perspective. A rainbow has two characteristics which speak volumes into that community. Gone were the colours black and white, quietly marginalized by the rainbow image. Gone too were confrontation, conflict and competition. In their place came harmony, joy and celebration, for a rainbow is about a whole enriched by the distinctiveness of the contrasting parts. This transformation was made possible by a great vision – the hope on which mourning and meekness are both built – incarnate in a person working to a costly higher agenda.

Though much remains to be done in South Africa, the name of Nelson Mandela will forever stand in that country as a symbol of a new beginning. Judging by the vast number of Mandela Streets, Avenues, Walks, Ways, Schools and Squares, across the nations of the world, he has indeed 'inherited the earth'!

MEANWHILE, IN OUR COMMUNITY ...

It is given to few of us to be involved in the writing of history on the scale of people like Vaclav Havel and Nelson Mandela, yet for us too this Beatitude can become a path on which to venture and a call that beckons us out of hiding.

It is a *call to care* about the world in which we live, whether the 'world' of our immediate family or household, or the 'world' of work, or the 'world' of this planet's delicate environment. That caring will begin for many of us by getting in touch with the pain and struggles of those worlds, facing rather than running from gaps between what is and what could or should be. It is the caring that refuses to settle for second best, the easy options or the false optimism that pass as substitutes for costly action.

It is *an invitation to join* in on an agenda that is already established and at work. It is the energizing power of the renewal of human society, which Christians recognize as the kingdom of God. This is where meekness calls us to listen and look for the vision of what could be, and then leave behind lesser hopes and visions.

It is a *vocation that shapes* who we are, as we dare to pour our energies into discerning and serving God's purposes in this world. It is this service of God that is not only true freedom, but the means through which we are shaped as people. It is in giving that we receive not only strength and wisdom for the task in hand, but greater affinity with God's generous nature.

... AND FINALLY

We need to note that the promise is not to *own* or possess the earth, but to *inherit* it. That means to receive it as gift. It is likely to mean the ability to enjoy and celebrate without the need to possess or control. It is not the way of the false prosperity gospel but the transformation of our whole mindset about owning, through the celebration of a world in some measure set free to be itself rather than mine.

Meditation

Blessed are the meek; for they will inherit the earth.
We come before you as those called to discern your will
We rejoice to share on earth the coming of your heavenly purposes

READING

> *Trust in the Lord and do good;*
> > *dwell in the land and enjoy safe pasture.*
> *Delight yourself in the Lord*
> > *and he will give you the desires of your heart.*
> *Commit your way to the Lord;*
> > *trust in him and he will do this:*
> *He will make your righteousness shine like the dawn,*
> *the justice of your cause like the noonday sun.*
> *Be still before the Lord and wait patiently for him;*
> > *do not fret when men succeed in their ways,*
> *when they carry out their wicked schemes.*
> > *But the meek will inherit the land*
> *and enjoy great peace.*
> (Psalm 37:1–7, 11)

HYMNS

> *Meekness and majesty,*
> > *manhood and deity,*
> *In perfect harmony,*
> > *the man who is God.*
> *Lord of eternity dwells in humanity,*
> *Kneels in humility and washes our feet*

O what a mystery,
    meekness and majesty.
Bow down and worship
    for this is your God.
This is your God.
Graham Kendrick

Will you come and follow me,
if I but call your name?
Will you go where you don't know,
and never be the same?
Will you let my love be shown,
will you let my name be known,
Will you let my life be grown
in you and you in me?
John L. Bell and Graham Maule

REFLECTION
    In what aspect of life is God calling us to wait for discernment of
        his purposes?
    Where, on earth, can we pray for revelation of God's purposes and
        the will to
        work with that higher agenda?

Blessed are the meek; for they will inherit the earth.

PRAYERS
    O Lord, we beseech you mercifully
        to hear the prayers
        of your people who call upon you;
    and grant that they may both perceive
        and know what things they ought to do,

and also may have grace and power
 faithfully to fulfil them;
through Jesus Christ your Son our Lord,
who is alive and reigns with you,
in the unity of the Holy Spirit,
one God, now for ever. Amen
Collect for the the 16th Sunday after Trinity

O Lord, from whom all good things come:
grant to us your humble servants,
that by your holy inspiration
we may think those things that are good,
and by your merciful guiding may
 perform the same;
through Jesus Christ,
who is alive and reigns with you,
in the unity of the Holy Spirit,
one God, now for ever. Amen
Collect for weekdays after Pentecost

Hungering and thirsting for righteousness does not mean

- preaching at people, moralizing or being judgemental and 'religious'
- a purely spiritual righteousness – personal rightness only
- an exclusive social action agenda – justice only.

Rather it is about ...

- desire for God's will – as the driving ambition of our lives
- right ordering of our lives as measured by God's purposes for us and the world
- sharing in God's passion for a just ordering of the world.

———————————

FIVE

SERVING YOU RIGHT

*Blessed are those who hunger and thirst for righteousness,
for they will be filled.*

Righteousness has never had a good press.

A few USA presidential elections ago, at the height of the Moral Majority movement, I heard a senator being interviewed in some current affairs programme in England. After talking about the impact of Moral Majority the interviewer then pointed out that scripture says 'when the righteous rule the land all will be well.' 'Yes,' said the senator, 'but just think what hell will be let loose when the self-righteous rule the land.' He expressed a widespread distaste for those who seek to moralize at us, preach at us, and take up a 'more righteous than you' stance.

One can trace this bad press right back to the Bible. The Pharisees were the classic exponents of a 'holier than thou' form of righteousness which Jesus challenges repeatedly in the Sermon on the Mount. The apostle Paul, himself formerly a Pharisee, expresses the typical wariness of people the world over towards this form of 'righteousness'.

Rarely will anyone die for a righteous person – though perhaps for a good person someone might actually dare to die. (Romans 5:7)

Long before Paul and the New Testament, righteousness had, arguably, no press at all. It was the great non-event of much religion. This was so, not because it was disliked, but rather because no one thought that righteousness (ethical and moral behaviour) had anything to do with religion, and with our relating to the supernatural forces around us.

One of the striking contributions of Moses, and the whole Jewish faith, to civilization was the strange and novel idea that religion and morality had anything to do with each other. Worship and ethics met on Mount Sinai. Maybe some people, realizing that Moses was making this strange connection – that how you behave matters to the god you worship – were saying to him, or at least thinking to themselves, 'This novel idea will never catch on.' Only it did, so much so that today we find it almost impossible to think of religion being unconnected to morality. We see it as the prime guardian and exponent of moral codes.

A DEFINING MOMENT

This bad press suggests that we need to clarify what we mean by the righteousness Jesus tells us we are hungering and thirsting after. Is there, in other words, a righteousness that can whet our appetite and create in us a desire for its enjoyment? My own experience led me to understand the nature of a desirable 'rightness' through a memorable, though painful experience.

One day on holiday, while in my late forties, I realized that I had stood on the water's edge at holiday time over two decades, watching with admiration the pleasure of windsurfers as they scudded, with such seeming ease, across the water. You could even say, at that stage, that I 'hungered and thirsted after' a go on a windsurfer. Realizing that time was running out, I took the plunge, paid up, and went for a two-hour lesson. We learned the theory first and then tried out our balancing skills with a board on the beach. It was designed to give us the feel of 'the real thing'.

Then came the great moment when the six of us were taken a little way out from the beach, allocated our boards and cut adrift. I actually did rather well. Indeed to this very day I can claim that I have never fallen off a surfboard. I climbed onto it and, with great trepidation, stood up. Then, with equal care – as if handling the most delicate and valuable piece of porcelain in the world – I pulled the sail up until I had a firm hold of the bar. The gentle wind, in so seemingly kind a way, gradually filled the sail and the board began to move. The feeling of elation was tinged only with a sense of trepidation. Gradually the trepidation increased as I headed towards a little bay about forty or fifty yards from the boat from which I had been set adrift. As I looked down at the sea around me I realized that I was now close in shore, in no more than two or three feet of water – and that I was surfing over a patch of rocks into which it would be foolish either to jump or fall backwards.

Warily I stepped backwards placing one foot on a carefully selected patch of sand between two rocky outcrops. My hands firmly gripped the bar of the sail and my other foot remained on the board, which continued to move, in a gentle arc, around the foot which by now was set like concrete in the wet sand below me.

Suddenly there was an ominous crack below me. Immediately I knew something serious had happened. I fell backwards onto the beach as the sailboard drifted away from me, out to sea. I never saw it, or got on another one, again. What I do remember – vividly – was lifting my left leg and seeing that my foot was facing out sideways, ninety degrees from its normal position. I nearly fainted at the sight. But I did not. Instead I started instinctively to look for help. There was not much of it about. It was a deserted beach, except for a boy about ten years old playing in the water twenty or more yards away from me. I began to call 'Help!' I saw him look at me two or three times and carry on with his game.

I realized why he seemed to lack any sense of urgency or compassion. When he looked, what he saw was a grown man with a wet suit on and an inflated life jacket, lying on the edge of the shore in less than one foot of water, with waves breaking no more than three or four inches high at the most. He hardly looked in urgent need of rescuing! Eventually curiosity got the better of him and he came over to me – even if only just to look. When I explained the problem and showed him my foot he went off to get his father, who rang for an ambulance.

In due course the ambulance arrived and took me off to hospital. Lying on a bed in the casualty department I heard two doctors talking about my situation. Their voices were low as was my consciousness. However, one phrase shouted out to me and brought me to full consciousness. I heard one say to the other something about a 'snatch re-set'. The word 'snatch' did not sound like good news. By now I was on full alert. One of them held down my thigh and began to explain what they were going to do ... when, without further warning, the other doctor 'did it'. He took firm hold of my foot, pulled it sharply down, swung it round and set it back in its socket!

It hurt!

I sat up holding my leg and found myself saying, 'Oh, ow, thank you; thank you, ow, oh' – repeatedly. Pain and pleasure were completely intermingled. The pain was real, but the pleasure and sense of relief in seeing my foot in the right place, was more real, more wonderful and more important. My foot was back in place, it had been put right, restored to its proper place and function. It felt wonderful. The relief was overwhelming!

I had experienced what righteousness is all about and found it to be good news. Righteousness is, quite simply, putting things right, restoring them to their full and intended purpose. It is essentially a matter of everything being put back into right relationship with the rest of creation which was originally intended for it.

———————————

God's judging does not mean an abstract, neutral, judicial act,
but an active, saving rearranging of broken relationships.

Duchrow and Liedke, *Shalom*

———————————

PROPHETIC RIGHTEOUSNESS

When Jesus uses the term 'righteousness' here in the Beatitudes it looks back to the prophets in the Old Testament. They continually challenged the children of Israel to practise righteousness in order that they might reflect the nature of God in their world. What the prophets were criticising was the people's preference for indulging in elaborate rituals, rather than in changing the way they lived. Typical of this prophetic call are the words of Isaiah:

Look, you serve your own interests on your fast days,
*   and oppress all your workers.*
Is such the fast that I would choose,
*   a day to humble oneself?*
Is not this the fast that I choose:
*   to loose the bonds of injustice,*
*   to undo the thongs of the yoke,*
to let the oppressed go free,
*   and to break every yoke?*
Is it not to share your bread with the hungry,
*   and bring the homeless person into your house;*
when you see the naked, to cover them,
*   and to hide yourself from your own kin?*
Then you shall call, and the Lord will answer;
*   you shall cry for help, and he will say, Here I am.*
(Isaiah 58:3, 5–7, 9)

God calls his people to a righteousness that acts on behalf of the poor and cares for distorted and destructive relationships – not only between people but in the way groups work – because this is what divine righteousness is about. Its focus is not on passing some 'piety exam' or 'respectability test' (though this is how the Pharisees had interpreted 'righteousness') but on sharing with God in bringing wholeness to every area of life. It is a righteousness active on behalf of others.

DESIRABLE RIGHTEOUSNESS

This is the righteousness at the heart of the attractiveness of Jesus Christ. 'The common people heard him gladly' because of his active concern for their welfare. He felt for, and acted on behalf of, those who were falling through the gaps of that society: the marginalized, poor, hungry, handicapped, unemployed and ostracized. To all he reached out with, literally, a helping hand; healing the sick, restoring the deranged, feeding the hungry. He did 'mind the gap', and moved to close it.

Even in his final confrontation with the religious and secular powers his goal was the same as in his work of forgiveness, acceptance and healing of individuals. He was out to set people free from forces within and beyond them that trapped, constrained and warped their lives. As he faced the full might of Roman and the religious powers, he was challenging those powers to give themselves to this higher agenda of God's renewing righteousness.

This is the righteousness of the broad canvas and of a whole-life perspective, a righteousness that belongs to the poor in spirit who recognize their need of partnership with and help from God and others. It is not a narrow religious righteousness that cannot see beyond the confines of church activity, but rather the passion for a world made whole. It embraces the world of personal morality and environmental concerns, the worlds of social justice and personal repentance, change and transformation, as well as the sheer creativity of community-building and artistic skills. All come together into the life-giving process that is at the heart of true righteousness.

The biblical understanding of righteousness fully integrates the personal and the social, the inner and the outer worlds. They become part of one single tapestry, woven together again and again. The description of the Suffering Servant in the prophecies of Isaiah expresses this integration of the personal and the public. It is a description of the interweaving of evangelizing the individual with the evangelizing of structures of injustice:

> *Here is my servant, whom I uphold,*
> *my chosen one in whom I delight;*
> *I will put my Spirit on him*
> *and he will bring justice to the nations.*
> *He will not shout or cry out,*
> *or raise his voice in the streets.*
> *A bruised reed he will not break,*
> *and a smouldering wick he will not snuff out.*
> *In faithfulness he will bring forth justice;*
> *he will not falter or be discouraged*
> *till he establishes justice on earth.*
> *In his law the islands will put their trust. (Isaiah 42:1–4)*

There is both gentle care for the bruised reed and strong assertion of the divine will in establishing justice on the earth. Both are evidenced in the life of Christ. He welcomes, affirms and gives honour and a place to the lame, the leper and the social outcasts; yet stands firm in challenging the abuse of power by the powerful. All too easily, we are strong with those to whom we feel superior (in skills, training, expertise) and deferential with those whom we judge to be more gifted, experienced and 'senior' to us. Jesus was gentle with the weak and strong before the powerful.

Moreover, he was continually working on the double agenda of meeting human needs at the personal level, and confronting injustices with the 'powers that be'. That double agenda came to its fullest expression in his entry into Jerusalem and his subsequent death at the hands of the unjust structures of power in church and society.

Righteousness, to put it another way, is a much stronger brew than simply personal morality. It is about that, but also about generous bias to the poor and courageous confrontation of injustice wherever it takes root.

LISTENING RIGHTEOUSNESS

This righteousness, which is at the heart of the ministry of Jesus, is no simple programme, or even set of principles, that once grasped can then be implemented by our own efforts. Rather it is a righteousness that reveals itself as you go; a righteousness that involves a listening ear more than anything else. Certainly Jesus was continually cautioning his disciples with that enigmatic phrase, 'He who has ears to hear, let him hear'.

Not that Jesus simply told others to listen; rather he modelled this as a central way of proceeding in his own life. It continued throughout his ministry.

The nights of prayer in which he engaged were about listening to the will of the Father. It was what was happening in his healing ministry. Those who desire to follow in the healing ministry today are often unconsciously frustrated by the sheer lack of pattern and technique in Jesus' healing work. Sometimes he spoke a word, and left it at that. At others he laid hands. For some he issued a challenge; for others he spat. No wonder people struggle to develop a technique out of that! The one consistent thing is that Jesus approached each situation with a fresh openness to God and the person and situation in front of him, and sought – in what today might be called 'listening prayer' – to discover the will of God.

The same approach is evident in Jesus' teaching or evangelistic ministry. It is difficult to discern any simple 'gospel outline' from what he says. To Zacchaeus he talks about hospitality, to the woman at the well about 'living water' and her 'home life', to the rich young ruler about possessions and to Nathanael about seeing him under a fig-tree. There is no simple technique in his personal, pastoral and evangelistic ministry. The common theme, however, is his evident listening to God and the needs of others in each situation he faces.

Such listening openness is itself a further demonstration of Jesus being poor in spirit. Not for him the assured technique or programme that needs to be implemented. Rather, the way he chooses is openness to God and human need coupled with discernment in every situation about the divine calling. That calling is in the direction of the restoration of every person and situation to their right relation to God, others and all creation.

Saints of all ages have made it their business to be present to God,
and out of this has sprung their truest vocation.

Leanne Payne, *The healing presence*

SATISFYING RIGHTEOUSNESS

The promise of this Beatitude looks as glaringly out of tune with our culture as the first part. Jesus pronounces as blessed those who seek God's will and way, the good of others and the well-being of the world around us. Such a way of life cuts right across the commitment to seek first our own security and advancement, and to 'do your own thing'. Our culture, the media and advertising, bombard us with such values every day: namely, that life is found in getting, and in getting more.

Yet Jesus quite specifically connects happiness, or satisfaction, with choosing this strange 'way of righteousness'. 'For they will be satisfied' is the promise. And it is quite a strong promise too. The word means 'stuffed full', 'filled to overflowing', satisfied above and beyond all expectations. Notice here that Jesus stays with the imagery of eating which is present in the first part of the Beatitude (hungering and thirsting). The conclusion is that a banquet awaits those willing to dare to live with this goal of righteousness as their heart's desire.

It is noteworthy how often Jesus used this feasting imagery in speaking about his own discovery of the will of God and his choosing to follow the Father's agenda for his life.

> One does not live by bread alone, but by every word that comes
> from the mouth of God. (Matthew 4:4)

> My food is to do the will of him who sent me and to complete his
> work. (John 4:34)

That is the promise of Christ, and the experience of many down the ages and across the globe. Whether working in an animal sanctuary, a two-thirds world literacy programme, a drop-in centre for the homeless, for the spread of faith in Christ, or proper protection of asylum seekers, their experience is that devoting ourselves to the service of others brings our own greatest fulfilment.

This sense of fulfilment is not restricted to involvement in projects alone. It is found in daily living in our close personal relationships, in our working (or lack of working) lives, and in our involvement in churches or communities. These are the primary spheres in which we are called to seek the agenda of righteousness. It is discovered as often as not in prayer and in conversation as (poor in spirit) we listen to others, care about what is missing (mourning), and wait (in meekness) to discern the higher agenda (hunger for righteousness). As we seek to do just that, the promise of God is that we will encounter God's presence in the process and – as the long-term consequence – know the satisfaction which engagement with the purposes of God alone can bring.

Choosing that higher, divine, agenda in the whole of our living will often be a costly and risky course. The promise of Christ is that it has a reward that nothing else can give. Why? Because we were made that way. We were made to be givers, because of what we have received. It is this truth that is expressed in those striking words of St Augustine when he spoke of God's service as perfect freedom. It is the freedom that is found on the path of those walking the way of righteousness.

Meditation

Blessed are those who hunger and thirst after righteousness, for they will be filled.
We come before you to discern and do your will
We rejoice that in your service is the fulfilment of our humanity

READINGS

Here is my servant, whom I uphold,
my chosen one in whom I delight;
I will put my Spirit on him
and he will bring justice to the nations.
He will not shout or cry out,
or raise his voice in the streets.
A bruised reed he will not break,
and a smouldering wick he will not snuff out.
In faithfulness he will bring forth justice;

he will not falter or be discouraged
till he establishes justice on earth.
In his law the islands will put their trust.
(Isaiah 42:1–4)

With what shall I come before the Lord
    and bow down before the exalted God?
He has showed you, O man, what is good.
    and what does the Lord require of you?
To act justly and to love mercy
    and to walk humbly with your God.
(Micah 6:6, 8)

HYMNS

Take my life, and let it be
    Consecrated, Lord, to thee;
Take my moments and my days,
    Let them flow in ceaseless praise.
Take my hands, and let them move
    At the impulse of thy love.
Take my feet, and let them be
    Swift and beautiful for thee.
Frances Ridley Havergal

Thy kingdom come, O God;
    Thy rule, O Christ, begin;
Break with thine iron rod
    The tyrannies of sin.

We pray thee, Lord, arise,
    And come in thy great might;
Revive our longing eyes,
    Which languish for thy sight.
L. Hensley

REFLECTION

Where is God calling us to discern and choose his way?

Where, on earth, should we pray for the coming of his kingdom of justice and mercy?

What part might we be called to play in the coming of that kingdom?

Blessed are those who hunger and thirst after righteousness, for they will be filled.

PRAYERS

O God,
who set before us the great hope
that your kingdom shall come on earth
and taught us to pray for its coming;
give us grace to discern the signs of its dawning
and to work for the perfect day
when the whole world shall reflect your glory;
through Jesus Christ our Lord. Amen
Celebrating Common Prayer, p. 68

Almighty God,
you have created the heavens and the earth
and made us in your own image:
teach us to discern your hand in all your works
and your likeness in all your children;
through Jesus Christ your Son our Lord,
who with you and the Holy Spirit
reigns supreme over all things,
now and for ever. Amen
Collect for the 2nd Sunday before Lent

SIX

PURPOSEFUL LIVING

*Blessed rather are those who hear the word of God
and obey it!*

Spirituality is one of today's buzz words. Everyone is 'into it' – even if many would be hard pressed to describe, let alone define it. It never was a very precise term, but the melting pot of modern society has added to the general confusion associated with its meaning. However, there is real value in looking at the Christian faith from the perspective of spirituality.

In reflecting on these last two Beatitudes (meekness and hungering for righteousness) it is helpful to consider what they have to say about the distinctive insights of Christian spirituality. Before doing this, however, we need to consider why spirituality is the track on which people are engaging with religion, faith and life today. Several things seem to be coming together here.

Materialism has created a desert. We have quite literally done that in the environment. By destroying vast rain forests – the lungs of planet Earth – at such an alarming rate we are creating new wildernesses. It is a picture of what is happening at the spiritual level. There is desert in the soul too. Possessions, security and status, image, acceptance and achievement, simply do not deliver the goods; of happiness, security or satisfaction. Like a person on a binge, we do not end up satisfied (as the fourth Beatitude promises); just sick. Material things in themselves do not address the spiritual depths of human nature. The search for the spiritual dimension in life seems to be a reaction to this materialism. 'There must be more to life than an upturn in the economy' is what this search is saying.

The famine in the West is far worse than that in the under-developed world for it is a famine of the spirit.

Mother Teresa of Calcutta

A fragmented world is looking for ways of putting life together again. The rational basis of modern culture has been brilliant in taking things apart. Splitting the atom is a classic illustration of this. However, what our society now hungers for is something that will put life back together again. Spirituality promises to do this, trying to make connections between my life, in all its fragmented 'bits', and some bigger, overall meaning and purpose in the universe. Spirituality is the search for meaning.

The loss of connection with Christianity which many people in the Western world experience means that people are looking elsewhere for spiritual resources. In some ways that is not surprising. Look at most Buddhist temples and you will see notices about prayer and meditation exercises and classes. Look at most church notice boards and you will find details of the next Fete, or Bring and Buy. Church notice boards give little indication that Christianity has any great connection with prayer, meditation or the spiritual dimension of life.

Yet spirituality is right at the heart of the Christian faith. Indeed, much of the transformation taking place in the church today is happening through the rediscovery of the spiritual roots of our Christian heritage. The faith is being reworked in the light of that rediscovery. The Retreat movement, Cursillo, Focolare and centres such as Lee Abbey, Iona and Taizé are all expressions of this shift.

Included in these signs of spiritual resurgence in the church is the Pentecostal and charismatic movement of this century. From a small prayer meeting in Azuza Street, Los Angeles, it has grown to embrace close on 250 million people across all continents. In the two-thirds world it usually combines striking corporate awareness of God with a strong thrust towards social transformation. Indeed many Pentecostal churches, for example in South America, would see 'speaking in tongues' as 'giving a voice to the voiceless'. In the West, the movement has been more vulnerable to emasculation through reduction to a privatized compartment of life disconnected from social engagement.

All these movements are evidences of spiritual vitality in the life of the church. As such they are a sign of the kingdom and manifestations of the presence of God at work today.

Spirituality connects with a privatized culture. In a world where the natural focus is on the individual, Christianity – or any other religion which expresses itself as 'organized religion' – may be at a disadvantage. Yes, there is a non-negotiable community dimension to the Christian faith and a dimension of social action; yet in an individualistic culture, we will have to learn how to start at the personal and individual and build up to the corporate and mission aspects. What is clear is that in such a privatized and individualized culture, connection with religion is taking place today most obviously through the practice of personal spirituality.

This was clearly illustrated in the response to the death of Diana, Princess of Wales. Despite the claims that we are a 'secular' culture, people in their millions instinctively looked for an expression of grief that was symbolic of some religious or spiritual dimension. There was a great sense of sharing together in a community in shock and grief, yet the outward form of corporate expression was that everyone did their own thing. People took flowers, which they bought, in their own time, to their own 'shrine' (and tens of thousands of them appeared virtually overnight). People put their own words in books of condolence, and stood at the gates of Kensington Palace or in churches or other places, in silence with their own thoughts. Here is corporate religion in a privatized culture.

So what does the Christian faith as a whole, specifically the Beatitudes and these two concerning meekness and righteousness in particular, tell us about what is distinctive in Christian spirituality? The following things stand out.

The great fact for which all religion stands is the confrontation of the human soul with the transcendent holiness of God.

John Baillie, *Our knowledge of God*

AN INTEGRATED SPIRITUALITY

None of the Beatitudes can be understood from within a privatized view of life or religion. They engage with the whole of life. The first two Beatitudes are about being in touch with the wonders, joys, surprises and the sorrow, struggles and injustices of our world. The second pair are about seeking to discover God's will in these situations. They are about being open to God's purposes in the world. Here is a spirituality that stays true to the whole of life.

This is in contrast to some spiritual practices, even within the Christian church, that focus on 'spirituality' as simply and exclusively a private and inner attitude. Such an approach can all too easily take us out of the world – on a permanent basis. Withdrawal, to be refreshed for new engagement with the whole of life, is one thing. Withdrawal, as a way of life, into a focus on private experiences of God, or into a narrowly defined 'spiritual compartment' in life, is another.

The incarnation of Christ is the root from which this integration grows. Christ, in his life, has shown us what it means to be engaged with the whole of life, the joys and struggles of our human existence and the whole created order. Any expression of the Christian faith, or of Christian 'spirituality', that permanently disconnects us from the sheer physical humanness of earthly existence, must therefore be named for what it is – sub-Christian at best.

One of the most shocking things about Jesus, and many of the saints, has been their proper love of life and of all creation. We see this in Jesus drawing endless lessons from the created order, in St Francis calling the moon 'brother moon' and in Mother Teresa seeing Christ in the face of the poor.

This refusal to compartmentalize faith or life is at the heart of true Christian spirituality. We need in our day particularly to hold on to this great gift of the Christian faith to touch the whole of human existence, and to resist the many pressures to privatize faith. It is one of the most precious gifts the Christian has to give to a fragmented world.

The greatest saints of God have been characterized, not by haloes and an atmosphere of distant unapproachability, but by their humanity. They have been intensely human and loveable people with a twinkle in their eyes.

James Philip, *Christian maturity*

A YIELDED SPIRITUALITY

Arguably *the* central distinctive of Christian spirituality is that it is focused outwards, not only on God in worship, but on the will of God – the coming of the kingdom – as the energizing focus for living. Much popular, and 'marketed', spirituality is concerned with helping me to get hold of spiritual power, for my own self-fulfilment and the enhancement of my personal well-being. In contrast, Christian spirituality finds its focus in the discovering and doing of the will of God. The concern of the Christian is not to gain power through prayer, but through prayer to yield ourselves to a Person.

It is this thrust of obedience that is at the heart of the meekness and hunger for righteousness of these two Beatitudes. It is about yielding to a higher agenda in seeking first the kingdom of God. This is a daring assertion, and personal discipline, in a culture structured around doing its own thing. The Christian is someone who not only prays, 'Your kingdom come', but seeks to live that way too.

There is a double sense in which the Christian is called to be eccentric. We normally use the word to describe someone whose actions and behaviour are different from the norm. As those called to live by faith in God, going the way of the cross, minding the gaps in life, and shaped by a vision of the coming kingdom, it is hardly surprising that we should sometimes be different. Not that being different is ever a healthy goal or aim, but it is likely to be the fruit of yielding to God's priorities. We may well be considered to be eccentric.

But there is another way in which discipleship calls us to be eccentric, because we are called to live with our centre outside ourselves – delighting in and devoting ourselves to the Beloved. This sort of eccentricity is what led Jesus to spend time in prayer, to be unafraid of the judgement of other people, and able to trust

God in the most testing of experiences. Yielded spirituality calls us to the same security of eccentric living.

The motivation and confidence to yield ourselves to God in this way comes through the practice of the first two Beatitudes. They lead us to experience God as loving, affirming and strengthening. Once that is our experience, trusting ourselves to God's will and God's way in our lives is a natural next step. Love turns obedience into an invitation.

We do not 'enjoy ourselves' in worship, indeed the very opposite ...
we cease to be absorbed by self and open out to God and his glory,
and our neighbour and his needs.

Forrester/McDonald/Tellini, *Encounter with God*

A TRANSFORMING SPIRITUALITY

Love is the power that transforms, because it invites our free co-operation with the process of transformation. Meekness is a trusting openness to God's purposes in our lives. Hungering and thirsting after righteousness is the expression of desire for the God who has met us in love, through Christ and by the Spirit. It expresses the response of love in desiring to join in with the purposes and concerns of the One who is loved.

This transformation takes place in a whole series of ways. *Our view of ourselves* is transformed because we discover we are loved by the God who made all that is and has created us to reflect something of his likeness in the world around. *Our view of the creation* is transformed: for we see it as made by God and made to fulfil his loving purposes. *Our view of others* is transformed: for we see God's image reflected in all other human beings. Moreover we also see other people as those through whom God speaks to and cares for us – giving love and affirmation and calling out our love and affirmation of others made in God's image.

This profound shift in how we see God, others, ourselves and the world around us is called conversion (literally 'turning around'). Though for some it begins as a single event, for every disciple it constitutes a way of life, a radical reordering of our lives around the purposes of God. The Greek word for conversion – *metanoia* – points to this 'about turn' for it means getting a new mind, one that takes us beyond our natural way of seeing and living life.

The apostle Paul describes the process and way of life in these illuminating terms:

> Do not be conformed to this world, but be transformed by the renewing of your minds, so that you may discern what is the will of God – what is good and acceptable and perfect. (Romans 12:2)

That change of mind, that new way of seeing life, inevitably leads to a changed lifestyle.

Falling, or being, in love is one of the best pictures of this process, for it speaks of a relationship which transforms our focus, priorities and the way in which we see and live life. For the disciples it meant leaving their boats and following Christ to become fishers of people rather than fishers of fish. For Francis of Assisi it meant leaving his aristocratic and wealthy background and wandering around the countryside as 'God's troubadour'. For many, such as Brother Lawrence, the transformation is in their attitude to an existing task, rather than changing of the task as such.

Just as lovers often adopt the interests of the one they love – *she* now cheering on his football team every week, whatever the weather: *he* discovering an interest in art he never knew he had, or even wanted! – so in discipleship. The transformation of life through the experience of God's love, and the response of loving attention, causes the disciple to order their life around God's 'interests'. And the divine interest is in the 'kingdom', the breaking in of God's loving purpose in the whole of human life. It is this that becomes the pearl of great price, and the 'one thing needed' which Mary chose. It is the transformation of desire, direction in life and in the way we live, reorientated around the coming of God's kingdom.

Evangelism is inviting people to respond to God's free and gracious invitation to be a part of his great mission to bring all things to a good End.

Robin Greenwood, *Practising community*

PURPOSEFUL LIVING

How does this Christian spirituality – that is, the Christian way of seeing and handling life – work out in practice if we live in the light of the Beatitudes? Three steps are important if we are to take this journey through life to which the Beatitudes call us.

Vision. This is where the journey begins. Certainly, hunger for God's perspective on life was the focus of Christ's life. It was, he said, his meat and drink to discover and do what the Father was showing him. Desire for God's way in his life was a major focus in his prayer life. It frequently preceded a new step forward in his ministry. Jesus continually engaged in prayer in order to review his priorities and focus. One of the occasions I love is recorded in Mark's gospel.

Very early in the morning, while it was still dark, Jesus got up, left the house and went off to a solitary place, where he prayed. Simon and his companions went to look for him, and when they found him, they exclaimed: 'Everyone is looking for you!' Jesus replied, 'Let us go somewhere else ...' (Mark 1:35–8)

This incident shows Jesus withdrawing after intense activity to listen to the Father, hungering after his will. As a result he emerges with a clear focus, and the inner strength to move forward and not be constrained by the expectation of others. It shows a wonderful sense of liberty from the pressures of life around him.

Hunger for a fresh vision of what God desires, in our personal and outward lives and in the life of the church, as well as in national and global events, is the source of vitality on which we are to draw. What motivates us, however, to engage in such prayer is the first two Beatitudes – being poor in spirit and mourning. If we think we have the answers to life we are not likely to look for them beyond our own inner resources. If we are content and satisfied with ourselves and the world around us, we are not likely to come in grief and longing before God. Being satisfied with what is cuts us off from the great good, and deeper satisfaction, God desires to impart. Comfortable Christianity saps the life out of discipleship.

Which is why prayer is the vital basis for all Christian action. But the prayer that Jesus modelled was not so much a 'God bless ...' approach, but rather a passionate personal desire for God himself, leading to a fresh insight to discern situations and discover what was pleasing to God. Without a similar hunger to know God and his will, our own ideas of what is right will crowd out any openness to the divine vision.

Vocation. Vocation arises out of vision. 'Vocation' is a concept sadly corrupted, even in the church, today. The most popular use of the word is to describe a few jobs – doctors, nurses, teachers and clergy. That is a travesty of the biblical understanding. The basic New Testament understanding of vocation is baptism – the call to discipleship. We cannot be followers of Christ without a vocation. But that vocation is not just about how we spend our working lives. Rather it is about living in response to the continually developing call of God. It is to be discerning, in the midst of daily living, as we handle ourselves and relate to those amongst whom we live and work.

This is true for churches also. They so easily lapse into no greater sense of direction than 'What shall we do for Lent this year?', when our real task is to discern God's will and agenda, not least when it cuts across received patterns or functions or personal or group preferences. Awareness of our own limitations and of the gap, in our life together and in the communities we are involved in, between what is and what God desires, gives urgency to this seeking after God's will. This gap is the fuel that energizes such prayer and can become the means of opening a faith community to the purposes of God.

If vision and vocation are not central to our living then we are likely to be 'driven' rather than 'called' people. When this happens we find ourselves at the mercy of events, frantically active yet seemingly going nowhere. Vocation gives a simplicity and focus that is both restful and purposeful. As Jesus put it:

> Come to me, all you that are weary and are carrying heavy burdens, and I will give you rest. Take my yoke upon you, and learn from me; for I am gentle and humble in heart, and you will find rest for your souls. For my yoke is easy, and my burden is light. (Matthew 11:28–30)

Choices. Those choices are usually about how to invest our time, energies, reputation, possessions and all that goes to make us who we are. It is in the choosing that we reveal and express the vision and the vocation that we have. Without this choosing our visions are no more than daydreams and vocation no more fruitful than wishful thinking. It is in the choosing and acting, and seeing things through, that fruit is borne from the inner convictions.

In a 'choice culture' it might be thought that this would come very naturally. However, our culture often pulls us away from choosing, for choosing one course precludes the option to follow another one. This is one of the distinctive contributions of the Christian faith to patterns of living – that choosing to follow our visions and vocation is how to live. Christ models this supremely for he accepted the limits of being born as one person, in one setting at one particular time. Yet his doing this made the truth that he revealed universal. It only becomes universal because it is first particular. So too for us. Choices that appear to restrict are actually what opens truth to us and those around us. Daring to choose God's way, and being willing to make sacrifices to that end, enable us to enter into purposeful living, shaped by meekness and a hunger after righteousness.

GIVING IT AWAY

How might this theme of purposeful living be expressed in the world around us – a world searching for values and purpose? Some steps we can take are as follows.

The higher agenda. Almost any activity or group, however great the initial vision, tends to lapse before long into 'keeping the show on the road', whether the 'show' is a marriage, family, voluntary project, school, church, business or government. It is vision that renews and can unite – if there is a widespread involvement in shaping the vision. An important role for Christians, seeking in their own lives to discover and do the will of God, is to help groups in which we are involved to come back regularly to addressing the basic question, 'What are we trying to do here?' In this way we can contribute to the refreshment of all engaged in the task through the recovery of shared vision.

The worthwhile sacrifice. Sacrifice, like obedience, is not a word that is used much today. Yet it is practised widely. There is no way of winning the World Cup (at anything), or climbing what we see as our 'mountain', or enjoying the creative arts, without sacrifice. Our heroes, whether pop stars or saints, are those who have made sacrifices for a particular end. Making sacrifices, and calling others to see the value of doing so (not as an end in themselves but as the means to achieving a higher agenda), is part of our service of the communities and groups in which we live. Finding ways of honouring those who make such sacrifices is one way of doing just this.

The good of all. We have seen that God's righteousness is about bringing all things into right relationship with each other. In view of this, the Christian has a particular calling to care for all involved in any venture. Organizations easily develop cultures in which one group gains at the expense of another. Sometimes a hospital or school seems to be run for the benefit of the staff rather than for the patients or pupils, or a business seems to be run for those at the top rather than for the benefit of all. The calling of the Christian is to work for ways in which all can benefit and in which all are cared for. This may not be an easy or popular path, but it is part of what it means to hunger after righteousness.

Purposeful living will stay close to the teaching and practice of Jesus in focusing on ways in which we can discern that presence of God in our world and share in his work of 'bringing all things to a good End'.

PART THREE:
Gracious living

Mercy does not mean

◆ pretending wrong does not matter
◆ never standing up to others
◆ taking the easy rather than the best way out of conflict.

Rather it is about ...

◆ giving to others – reckless generosity (like God's)
◆ forgiveness: releasing others from their debts
◆ seeking what is best for others, even at cost to ourselves
◆ overcoming evil with good rather than 'retaliating in kind'.

───────────────────

SEVEN

GIVING AS GOOD AS YOU GET

Blessed are the merciful,
for they will receive mercy.

A friend of mine was recently at a refugee camp in Africa. It was a vast complex of over fifty thousand people representing eleven different nationalities. She was visiting the Sudanese community (twenty-three thousand people), the vast majority of whom were Christians. It was a scene of almost unimaginable suffering and poverty that greeted her. Many of those in the camp had been there for over six years with seemingly no hope of returning home in the foreseeable future.

At one stage she met with a group of the women who, with strong passion and much finger-wagging, spoke to her of the sense of injustice they felt at being forgotten by the outside world. At the end of the meeting they took her to the hut where she was to sleep – and washed her feet! Here was no docile abandonment of hope or submissive yielding to hopeless events. Rather there was passionate expression of righteousness, which yet led straight into an act of mercy.

This experience was underlined in a different way when she was asked to address a group of women from the camp and speak 'a word from God' to them. Wrestling with what she might say, she could not see anything to say about their outward circumstances. Rather, she chose to address the inner strength that God gives which enables us to 'keep faith' in the most testing of life circumstances. Using Paul's prayer in Ephesians, namely: 'I pray that, according to the riches of his glory, you may be strengthened in your inner being with power through the Spirit' (Ephesians 3:16), she pointed them to the grace of God. That prayer, incidentally, is close to the thrust of the first four Beatitudes which describe the journey we need to make if we are to cope with the pain, struggles and limitations of our earthly existence and come through to a desire for the things of God.

At the end of her talk the women then said they had a verse to give to her. It was Matthew 5:7–9 – these next three Beatitudes with their call to be merciful, pure in heart and peacemakers. It was a word to the West about the actions we can take on behalf of the powerless wherever they live.

What mercy glimpses is the whole world made new.

Simon Tugwell, *The Beatitudes*

HOLY MOSES

In looking at righteousness in the fourth Beatitude we considered Moses, who had previously only known an anger that consumed. At the burning bush he discovered a righteousness and passion for justice that brought life and freedom to the children of Israel. But how did he get there? Well, it was a journey; a long and tortuous one that took him over forty years to complete. It took him to the land of Midian; a land where he felt deeply estrangement, longing to be back with 'his' people. The name he gives to his first child tells it all:

He named him Gershom: for he said, 'I have been an alien residing in a foreign land.' (Exodus 2:22)

He is acutely aware of his distance from all that means 'home' to him. He has not settled but remains restless in spirit. He is here expressing his experience of being *poor in spirit*. It was this sense of poverty, powerlessness and failure that had prompted him to flee from Pharaoh – for he knew he was no longer acceptable either in Pharaoh's court or amongst the Israelite community.

The name given to his son expresses his deep sense of alienation. He is cut off from his people – and it hurts. He certainly does 'mind the gap': he is *mourning*. Yet he stays. He has learned a proper *meekness* and knows that taking the law into his own hands again is not an option open to him. So the naming of his son may well also be a prayer; that the day will come when the distance is closed and he is once again part of his own people. It may well be that openness to what God may yet plan for him (*hungering after righteousness*) prompts him instinctively to pay attention to this burning bush.

In other words, Moses' life can be seen as a journey through the Beatitudes.

However, we need to be careful of the picture of a journey. Where it breaks down is that it can be taken to imply that being poor in spirit, mourning, meek or any of the other Beatitudes, may simply be a 'passing phase' – with the implication that we will 'grow out of it'. They are not like that. The Beatitudes are something we grow into, not out of. In that sense they are more like a building, for the initial Beatitudes are foundations on which we build. As such they are essential to the upholding (literally the 'holding up') of the superstructure which then emerges.

THE MEANING OF MERCY

If righteousness has a bad press, mercy suffers from an almost complete lack of press. Rarely do TV news or national newspapers tell a story about mercy. Scandal, failure, greed, immorality have guaranteed publicity. There seems to be a privacy law at work when it comes to mercy. News of its presence rarely seeps out. But it is there all the same; though it has a strong preference for undercover, rather than overt, operations.

I think of a woman priest whose small congregation of 25 were all expected to be present for *the* major service of the year – a communion service on Easter Sunday. But when the great day arrived only 22 turned up. The priest was really upset. Had so little of the faith got through to these members of the church that they had not seen the priority of this Easter celebration? They had been at the service on Good Friday, she knew they were not away for the weekend, so why were they absent? Three days later, she stumbled across the answer.

She found the three at the home of a dying member of the community; and they were evidently not just visiting but living there. She then discovered that, in response to the Good Friday service, and the meditation on the women at the foot of the cross of Christ, these three women had sensed God calling them to move in with the dying woman and give her the constant support and help she needed.

The woman died three weeks later. Just before she died, she said to the woman priest, 'The last three weeks have been the most wonderful three weeks of my life, I have never felt so loved.' She had experienced mercy.

Mercy comes as such a surprise at this point of the Beatitudes if the analysis of the overarching pattern is right, for who of us would identify mercy as the first mark of righteousness? Righteousness is seen as censorious, strident, judging and, too often, what we think other people should do. Mercy is seen, rather like meekness, as weak and insipid, with a touch of saying, 'There, there, everything will be all right.' But righteousness is not like that: it is a passion to put things right bound up with a willingness to be involved in making sacrifices to that end. Equally mercy is not like its popular caricature; it is a strong and energetic commitment to seeing right done so that all may share in our experience of the grace and generosity of God.

Mercy is the outpouring to others of God's gift of mercy that we have experienced.

Michael Crosby, *Spirituality of the Beatitudes*

THE MERCIFUL CHRIST

One of the best ways to see what mercy means is to look at the actions of Jesus immediately after the preaching of the Sermon on the Mount. First he heals a leper, then he welcomes and affirms the faith of a Roman centurion, and then he heals Peter's mother-in-law and a multitude of other, unnamed, people. Here is mercy, or righteousness, in action.

It is about affirming (literally 'making strong') those who are socially outcast and physically weak. It is also about active goodness, going out of our way to put good into a situation and into the life of another human being.

It certainly seems to include stepping out of the framework of normal social conventions and touching the untouchables (the leper), holding conversation with someone who was definitely not 'one of us' (the centurion), and generously reaching out to people (the multitude) not considered worth caring about.

This link between mercy and righteousness can be traced back to the Old Testament and to the oft-repeated refrain of 'justice, mercy and the knowledge of God'. The whole law of Moses is built around those three pillars. Justice, doing what is right; mercy, counting others in; and the knowledge of God, as the goal of righteousness and mercy.

Again we see the strength of mercy here, as we saw the strength of meekness earlier, for it includes not simply giving to the needy, but continually challenging and renewing the structures of society to count those outside in, and to include the poor and needy in the total distribution of wealth. This costly redistribution is not just a matter of hand-outs, but includes structures of justice which give an equal share of available resources so that everyone can 'make their own way in life'.

The whole of Jesus' ministry can be seen in this light. He came to demonstrate the merciful nature of God's righteousness. Twice Jesus quotes Hosea: 'I desire mercy not sacrifice' (Matthew 9:13, 12:7) He then adds, 'Go and learn what this means', which suggests that the natural person does not immediately think or act this way.

He drew a circle
that shut me out.
Heretic, rebel,
a thing to flout!
But love and I had
the wit to win;
we drew a circle
that took him in.

Edwin Markham

PRACTISING MERCY

What mercy means for us can be grasped by recapturing the original sense of a number of phrases we use in popular speech today but which are taken in a cynical and negative way.

Putting them right. This saying takes us back to the link between righteousness and mercy. Mercy is the first step in the application of righteousness. It is about restoring the harmony, balance and order of all creation, of human society and relationships, and of the inner being of each individual.

It is this 'putting right' which we see in Jesus' action towards the leper and the centurion. He is affirming their worth and dealing with their different estrangements from the community around them. It is a social, spiritual, emotional, physical and political action that Jesus is involved in. It is that same all-embracing generosity and goodness to others that is the character of God which is being built into the children of the kingdom, making us channels of overflowing (in fact, recycled) generosity.

Giving as good as you get. We use this phrase to express our desire, or advice to someone, to make life difficult for others. Mercy is rather about doing good to others and giving them what is needed for their fuller experience of life. Mercy is part of a 'virtuous spiral' or current of grace. As we come to recognize God's goodness and generosity, forgiveness and delight towards us, it becomes the fuel on which our own self-worth and self-acceptance run. We are then able to give as good as God gives to us. The promise built into this Beatitude then completes the cycle – 'for they will receive mercy'. It points to the truth expressed elsewhere by Jesus that the measure we use in giving to others is the one which will be used for us. If we give a thimbleful of generosity to others, that thimble will be the measure for what God gives to us.

If, on the other hand, we use a bath as our measure of mercy, we will find ourselves immersed in it, cleansed by it, and ourselves refreshed.

Repaying them in kind. The currency that the follower of Christ has become familiar with is 'the goodness and loving kindness of God'. We are therefore able to give out of the store of grace, rather than out of retaliation. A little boy recently stated in an examination paper that 'Jesus Christ gave us the Golden Rule – to do one to others before they do one to you'! You can see how he got there. He began, no doubt, with the words 'Do unto others', but then realized that that could not be right. There is no such word as 'unto', at least not in his vocabulary. So it must be 'one to'. However, once you begin by saying 'Do one to others ...' the culture around tells you what the second half of the sentence must be.

Putting them in their place. Jesus was continually putting people in their place. Back in the homes from which they had been sent away – such as lepers, the blind and beggars. Back in the community from which their own actions had cut them off – such as Zacchaeus. Back in touch with right sexual relationships – the woman of Samaria and the woman caught in adultery, and the men who had been eager to judge that woman. Back in touch with God – Nicodemus, the disciples and the multitudes. Back in touch with the limits of their power and in touch with their God-given responsibilities – Pilate and the religious leaders. Back in touch with their loved ones – by healing the sick and raising the dead.

Serving them right. This is the continual experience of people who give to others on the margins of society. Many who are involved in ventures such as Samaritans, the Hospice movement and Cruse speak about the blessing it is to them and of all that they receive from those whom they are seen as 'serving'. Those who serve the poor are most aware of what they receive, rather than give, to such people. How true it is that although the poor need the church and others, it is even more true that we, the church, need the poor. It is they who put life in perspective and seem continually able to be a blessing to us.

Is it not striking that our culture has so many terms which, on the face of it, sound positive yet which by common use have become negative, hostile and destructive? The calling of Christians may not include rescuing the language. It certainly does involve reviving the practices to which these phrases point, when rightly understood.

Choosing the way of Christ and restoring these popular sayings to their original meaning is costly. Counting others in rarely happens without putting ourselves out.

Next to the Blessed Sacrament itself, your neighbour
is the holiest object presented to your senses.

C. S. Lewis, *The weight of glory*

A NEW AND LIVING WAY

There are two natural responses to danger: fight or flight. We hit out or make a run for it; literally or emotionally. Jesus shows us a third way: the way of mercy. This is the way of generous engagement with what may well be threatening.

We see retaliation in all the major trouble spots of the world. We can begin the process of reversing this trend by praying for those who oppose, offend, or stand for something contrary to us. It must begin with prayer, for that is where we are often first made aware of the mercy we have received. But mercy cannot stop at prayer. Merciful praying leads to a merciful attitude and on to merciful action. Where it does not, the flow of mercy is being blocked. 'Being perfect' means being 'merciful' like the One we worship. He has been revealed to us as the One who acts in mercy.

Not that this means pretending everything is wonderful or that no one is ever capable, or culpable, of doing wrong. But it is about seeing beyond the wrong to what can be, and contributing into that situation out of all the goodness and mercy that we have received.

How much our world needs a vast army of people who, having resisted the temptations of flight or fight, have chosen the third way of merciful righteousness.

Meditation

Blessed are the merciful, for they will receive mercy.
We come before you thankful for your ceaseless goodness towards us
We rejoice to join with you in sharing that goodness even to our enemies

READINGS
Prayerful mercy

You have heard that it was said, 'You shall love your neighbour and hate your enemy.' But I say to you, Love your enemy and pray for those who persecute you, so that you may be children of your Father in heaven: for he makes his sun rise on the evil and on the good, and sends rain on righteous and on the unrighteous. For if you love those who love you, what reward do you have? Do not even tax collectors do the same? And if you greet only your brothers and sisters, what more are you doing than others? Do not even the Gentiles do the same? Be perfect, therefore, as your heavenly Father is perfect. (Matthew 5:43–8)

Merciful action

With what shall I come before the Lord
and bow myself before God on high?
Shall I come before him with burnt offerings,
with calves a year old?
Will the Lord be pleased with thousands of rams,
with ten thousands of rivers of oil?
Shall I give my first born for my transgression,
the fruit of my body for the sin of my soul?
He has told you, O mortal, what is good
and what does the Lord require of you.
but to do justice, and to love kindness
and to walk humbly with your God?

(Micah 6:6–8)

HYMN

When all thy mercies, O my God,
My rising soul surveys,
Transported with the view, I'm lost
In wonder, love and praise.

A heart in every thought renewed,
And full of love divine:
Perfect and right and pure and good –
A copy, Lord, of thine!
Joseph Addison

REFLECTION

Who are my enemies – people I find most difficult to get on with – for
whom I should pray?
Where is God calling us to act mercifully, in a way I would want to be
treated if I found myself in similar circumstances?

What part can we play in working for merciful structures wherever people work together?

Blessed are the merciful, for they will receive mercy.

PRAYERS

O God, you declare your almighty power
most chiefly in showing mercy and pity:
mercifully grant to us such a measure of your grace,
that we, running the way of your commandments,
may receive your gracious promises,
and be made partakers of your heavenly treasure;
through Jesus Christ your Son our Lord,
who is alive and reigns with you,
in the unity of the Holy Spirit,
one God, now and for ever. Amen
Collect for the 11th Sunday after Trinity

Almighty God,
who sent your Holy Spirit
to be the life and light of your Church:
open our hearts to the riches of your grace,
that we may bring forth the fruit of the Spirit
in love and joy and peace;
through Jesus Christ your Son our Lord,
who is alive and reigns with you,
in the unity of the Holy Spirit,
one God, now and for ever. Amen
Collect for the 9th Sunday after Trinity

Purity of heart does not mean

- never recognizing wrong-doing, or naming it as such
- being 'so heavenly minded that we are no earthly use'
- only ever saying nice (and sugary) things about life, the world and others
- being too good to be true; rather it is about being true to what is good.

Rather it is about ...

- seeing through things – to their true meaning, purpose and relationship to God
- seeing beyond the immediate and obvious to God and his purposes in every situation
- the vision of the artist to see how often lifeless material can be given life and meaning
- an honesty about ourselves that results in generosity towards others

EIGHT

SEEING STRAIGHT

Blessed are the pure in heart,
for they will see God.

The story is told of a meeting between the scientist Albert Einstein and the prominent psychologist C. G. Jung. Jung was asking Einstein how long it had taken him to work out his theory of relativity and indicating that it must have involved years of exhausting mental effort. 'Oh, no,' said Einstein. 'The figures just danced before my eyes, all I had to do was work out what they meant.' He saw in a moment. What took the time was working out what it all meant.

Michelangelo, the painter and sculptor, was asked how he set about carving his great masterpieces like *David* or *Moses*, when faced with a formless mass of stone. He said that he saw them in the stone 'crying out to be released'. Where no one else could see anything but stone, Michangelo saw a finished sculpture.

One of England's greatest landscape artists, Turner, was at an exhibition of his paintings when someone came up to him and said, 'I don't see clouds and water like that, Mr Turner.' The artist replied, 'But don't you wish you could?!' It was a wonderful reply from someone who had seen something of the uniquely English nature of the landscape around him, and had been able to capture it on canvas.

All three of those stories are about seeing. But they are more than about simply seeing things physically present. We can 'see' someone's emotions by their body language, we can see their response to our invitation by looking at their face, well ahead of their saying anything. But seeing has an element of revelation about it too. 'Ah, yes, now I see.' It may be one of those magic-eye three-dimensional pictures that you have to look at in an unfocused way, or trying to find out where a leak in the plumbing is, or wanting to understanding why someone looked so puzzled when you said something. Suddenly we 'see' it – and say, 'It's so obvious now.'

It is this *seeing through* that is at the heart of this Beatitude. It is about seeing through to the heart of the issue. It is something that all of us long for, whether we call it a sixth sense or say, as all of us have done at various points in our lives, 'If only I had seen.' 'It was staring me in the face, but I did not recognize it,' we say with hindsight (notice how that word also uses the idea of seeing).

---

*Beauty is the real aspect of things when seen aright
and with the eyes of love.*

Kathleen Raine

IS PURITY OUT OF ORDER?

At first sight (note again the all-pervasive imagery), it looks as if this Beatitude does not fit into the flow of them all. Particularly is this so if you accept the earlier argument that the three Beatitudes, mercy, purity of heart and peacemaking, are about the practice of righteousness. Purity of heart does not seem to be about any sort of 'practice'. It is essentially a private, even hidden work. Which is just why it fits. It is about the inner stillness, waiting and discernment that are at the heart of true justice, righteousness and the coming of God's kingdom. Purity of heart puts our own motives, assumptions and expectations in order, so that we may be part of the solution in the situations around us, rather than part of the problem itself.

It points us to the focus on God and God's will that moved Jesus, in the midst of a hectic schedule, to spend time in prayer. In prayer he gained a new insight – for example, about what to do next, which disciples to choose, why Jerusalem should be his destination and what was going to happen there. In prayer, Jesus saw the way ahead.

Not that he stopped for a prayer meeting every time difficult situations faced him. Rather, his previous stillness before the Father prepared him to see through to the heart of situations, in the midst of life, as he faced difficult choices.

So purity of heart brings a proper order to the various emotions, options and responses that stir within us. Without this clarity of vision, justice cannot be done. Indeed justice cannot be seen, let alone seen to be done. And justice requires a whole range of responses in different situations. Jesus, confronted by a disturbed man in a synagogue, 'sees' not only the demonic forces at work in him, but also what was in the heart of the scribes and Pharisees as they looked for some grounds to accuse him of being a sabbath breaker. Purity of heart frequently led Jesus to confront injustice, unmask hypocrisy and challenge hidden motivation in those around him. It was certainly not synthetic sweetness.

So, for us to act in righteousness (the fourth Beatitude), our first step is one of mercy (the fifth Beatitude), followed as quickly as possible by one of revelation, insight, discernment to see through to the heart of the issue, to see 'what is really going on here' and thus what the situation requires (this sixth Beatitude).

IF LOOKS COULD KILL!

Seeing straight does not come easily or naturally to us human beings. We are continually only seeing part of the picture, drawing wrong conclusions or missing the important things. We often see only what we expect to see.

Jesus, in the Sermon on the Mount, traces much human distress back to this failure to see straight. He speaks about the lustful look as one that is abusive of others and also to the one who looks. This is not about rejecting the attractiveness of the opposite sex but rather about indulging in the fantasy that makes another person into an object. It is about the distorted vision of seeing someone as 'something'; and then imagining 'using' this other person as a thing. The pure in heart can see the beauty – yes, including the sexual beauty – of another human being, without turning it into lust.

Later on in the Sermon, Jesus uses another of his graphic pictures (which help us 'see truth'), when he says:

> Do not judge, so that you may not be judged. For with the judgment you make you will be judged, and the measure you give will be the measure you get. Why do you see the speck in your neighbour's eye, but do not notice the log in your own eye? Or how can you say to your neighbour, 'Let me take the speck out of your eye,' while the log is in your own eye? You hypocrite, first take the log out of your own eye, and then you will see clearly to take the speck out of your neighbour's eye. (Matthew 7:1–5)

Notice how strongly the metaphor of sight figures here. It is all about getting things out of our eyes. Notice also the link with mercy: 'the measure you give will be the measure you get'. Which is why *how* we see is so important. Righteousness cannot be advanced, mercy expressed or justice done, if our seeing is distorted. So we need to pay attention to how we see.

Purity of heart clarifies vision.
Simon Tugwell, *The Beatitudes*

SEEING EYE TO EYE WITH GOD

One of the finest and most extensive treatments of this theme of purity of heart is the vision (the 'seeing' imagery, again) of Isaiah in the Temple:

> In the year that king Uzziah died, I saw the Lord sitting upon a throne, high and lofty; and the hem of his robe filled the temple. Seraphs were in attendance above him; each had six wings; with two they covered their faces, and with two they covered their feet, and with two they flew. And one called to another and said:
> 'Holy, holy, holy is the Lord of hosts:
> the whole world is full of his glory.'
> The pivots on the thresholds shook at the voices of those who called, and the house was filled with smoke. And I said: 'Woe is me! I am lost, for I am a man of unclean lips, and I live among a people of unclean lips; and yet my eyes have seen the King, the Lord of hosts!'
> Then one of the seraphs flew to me, holding a live coal that had been taken from the altar with a pair of tongs. The seraph touched my mouth with it and said: 'Now that this has touched your lips, your guilt has departed and your sin is blotted out.' Then I heard the voice of the Lord saying, 'Whom shall I send, and who will go for us?' And I said, 'Here am I; send me!' (Isaiah 6:1–8)

The death of king Uzziah had been a cruel blow to the young prophet, for the king had been a godly reformer who began his reign by bringing about a series of changes that came under that Old Testament description of 'doing that which was right in the sight of God'. He was the John F. Kennedy of his day, the young, visionary leader who would bring about change for the better and whose very presence on the scene gave hope to all.

Then, as so often happens with visionary reformers, arrogance crept in and he thought he could do no wrong. One day he entered the temple and offered the sacrifice, which only the priests were allowed to do. He had stepped over the line drawn by God between king and priest. He had taken the law into his own hands and brought down upon himself the judgement of God. He became a leper and shortly afterwards he died.

It was in the vacuum left by his death and his moral crusade, that Isaiah came into the Temple. No doubt he hoped to 'hear' from God in some way. What happened was that he saw – a vision. It was a vision of God filling the temple, his whole world at that moment. Where, before, he had 'seen' darkness and no shape to the future, a political 'black hole', now he found this brilliance of revelation which reminded him that his faith needed to be in the God of Uzziah, not in Uzziah as god.

The seeing not only took him to the realms of heaven, in this great 'heavenly vision', but also took him on a journey within. It was a painful journey into the darkness of his own heart, and of the community around him. 'I am lost, for I am a man of unclean lips, and I live among a people of unclean lips; and yet my eyes have seen the King, the Lord of hosts!'

This second stage of seeing (that is, seeing himself and the nation in their true colours before God) leads into an experience of cleansing. Fire from the altar – another symbol of purity – touches his lips in a cleansing act. His seeing turns now to hearing the call of God for the work that is to be done: 'Then I heard the voice of the Lord saying, "Whom shall I send, and who will go for us?" And I said, "Here am I; send me!"'

---

*It is in learning how to see things properly that we first begin
to be enchanted by the beauty of God.*

Origen

ISAIAH AND THE BEATITUDES

One of the striking aspects of this story is the way that the journey
of the Beatitudes is evident in the prophet's experience.

Isaiah enters the Temple in great *poverty of spirit*. Perhaps
today we would say he felt 'gutted'. Though he may have felt he
did not know 'which way to turn', he instinctively turns towards
the Temple, and the place of meeting with God. He knows he
needs help from beyond himself. He is at the end of his resources –
and the beginning of God's.

He is in *mourning*, and not only for the king but for the nation
too. As the vision breaks in upon him it deepens this sense of
mourning, this gap between the holiness of God and the unclean-
ness of people. Indeed this grief about sin engulfs him too. 'Woe is
me' is his first response to this vision. Here is no comfortable 'feel-
good' vision or experience, but one that purges him and addresses
the real weakness and brokenness in him and the people.

There is a marvellous Peanuts cartoon of Charlie Brown in bed
saying 'Sometimes I lie awake at night and ask myself, "Where
have I gone wrong?"' In the second picture he is still there and
says, 'Then I hear a voice saying, "This is going to take more than
one night!"' It is a wonderful reminder that seeing is not only difficult, a skill and disposition we need to learn, but is often also a
painful experience; for it is facing reality.

The whole process is about a proper sense of *meekness* and of hungering for *righteousness*. The prophet longs to discover God in the mess that is all around him. In that openness to God, and the willingness to wait in order to discern the purposes of God, the first thing that hits him is the *mercy* of God. The coals from the altar do not consume him, but rather cleanse him and set him free to be of service in the purposes of God. Here again, as with the burning bush and the tongues of fire at Pentecost, is fire that purifies but does not consume.

The coals *purify* his vision, first of himself and then of the nation and his calling to serve his people. That cleansed way of seeing results in his hearing the call of God to be part of the divine *peacemaking* agenda in a broken society. The outcome, as the rarely read second half of the chapter makes clear, is *persecution*. More on that in the chapter on the last Beatitude.

SEEING THINGS THROUGH

Seeing aright is the essential requirement if we are to do right or put things right; which is why purity of heart is foundational to true righteousness. So the final question which this Beatitude raises for us is about how we can see like this. How can we gain the vision we need so as to participate in God's purposes in the whole of our living? The following steps have proved to be crucial in the experience of the saints down the ages.

Honesty about our own motivation is a vital starting point. The most dangerous hidden agendas are the ones that are hidden in our own hearts, which is why the practice of confession, whether as a sacramental act or part of a personal spiritual discipline, is basic to holiness. The prayer of Psalm 51 – indeed the whole psalm is a classic text on repentance – is:

You desire truth in the inward being;
    therefore teach me wisdom in my secret heart ...
Create in me a clean heart, O God,
    and put a right spirit within me. (Psalm 51:6, 10)

Being open to new possibilities is the next step. Sometimes we can have too much experience. 'That will never work', 'They never do a decent job', 'I've tried that before', all too easily spring to our lips. What we need to look for is a fresh angle on a difficult or resistant situation, or fresh hope about someone who concerns us. This means submitting our thoughts to God in prayer. The idea of 'submitting' thoughts to God in prayer suggests the practice of 'submitting a report'. When we do that, we expect a response. It may be one of affirmation ('You are on the right lines'), or correction ('Why no mention of ...?') or of alerting us to new possibilities ('Have you thought about ...?'). In this process, our ideas are reshaped. Another aspect of submitting our thoughts to God in prayer is the willingness to let go our limited vision in order to discover God's purposes. Prayer is a vital part of seeing through to God's answers.

Being shaped by the truth. Our vision is shaped by what we see, and by what we allow to shape our innermost thoughts. The Anglican principle about liturgy is that 'the word spoken is the word believed'. Truths laid down deep in our memory can shape the way we see life. Taking time for meditation on the truth can, little by little, as part of a lifetime's discipline, help to shape our way of seeing life. Meditation is the practice of turning the truth over in our minds again and again, until its reality comes alive to us. Facing a difficult situation where we do not see what to do, it can be helpful to repeat quietly to ourselves a scripture passage such as this Beatitude – *blessed are the pure in heart, for they will see God.* We can then repeat it slowly, adding a brief one-sentence thought or prayer between each repetition – such as

♦ what does purity of heart mean in this situation?
♦ where can I see God at work here?
♦ what is really going on here?
♦ what good can come out of this experience?

How you see the problem is the problem.

Anon.

Dreaming dreams. Dreams and visions go hand in hand in scripture and Christian spiritual tradition. They are about seeing the future. The three stories with which this chapter opened were about people seeing things that would shape the future in different ways. The Christian virtue of hope is about believing that there will be a way through and so looking for it.

Not that such dreams are necessarily always found in prayer and meditation. They can just as likely be found in the midst of faithful action. Mother Teresa spoke of seeing Christ in the face of the poor. It is this that is the basis of the final judgement, which itself is nothing other than the final unveiling, the Final Seeing. Jesus spoke of that finale as being worked out in the present in such a way that these two Beatitudes of being merciful and pure in heart are seen as one, when he said: 'Just as you did it to one of the least of these who are members of my family, you did it to me.'

This purity of heart is what enables us to see the purposes of God in our lives, and in so doing to be touched by the holiness, mercy and generosity of God himself. In such seeing, we see through to the love at the heart of the universe, to God himself. But it does not happen automatically. Rather, in the midst of daily living, God calls us to choose purity of heart in order that we may see His way, choose his attitudes, and discover Him for his own sake at the heart of all our merciful and righteous living.

Meditation

Blessed are the pure in heart, for they will see God.
We come before you so that we may see all life through your eyes
We rejoice in the beauty, even in its brokenness, of all that you have made

READINGS

> *O God, you are my God, I seek you,*
>   *my soul thirsts for you;*
> *my flesh faints for you,*
>   *as in a dry and weary land*
>   *where there is no water.*
> *So I have looked upon you in the sanctuary,*
>   *beholding your power and glory.*
> *Because your steadfast love is better than life,*
>   *my lips will praise you.*
> *So I will bless you as long as I live*
>   *I will lift up my hands and call*
>   *on your name.*
>
> (Psalm 63)

If you know that he is righteous, you may be sure that everyone who dies right has been born of him. See what love the Father has given us, that we should be called children of God; and that is what we are. The reason the world does not know us is that it did not know him. Beloved, we are God's children now; what we will be has not yet been revealed. What we do know is this: when he is revealed, we will be like him, for we will see him as he is. And all who have this hope in him purify themselves, just as he is pure.

(1 John 2:29–3:3)

HYMNS

> *Blest are the pure in heart,*
> *For they shall see our God;*
> *The secret of the Lord is theirs,*
> *Their soul is Christ's abode.*
> John Keble

> *For the beauty of the earth,*
> *For the beauty of the skies,*
> *For the love which from our birth*
> *Over and around us lies,*
> *Lord of all, to thee we raise*
> *This our grateful hymn of praise.*
> F Sandford Pierpoint

REFLECTION

> *What situation do I face at present where I need to gain a fresh insight*
> *of how God sees what is happening, or failing to happen?*
> *Where, in the world, do we need to pray that all involved will be given*
> *purity of heart?*
> *What might either my immediate situation, or the global need, look*
> *like if we could see it from God's perspective?*

Blessed are the pure in heart, for they will see God.

PRAYERS

> *Almighty God,*
> *to whom all hearts are open,*
> *all desires known*
> *and from whom no secrets are hidden:*
> *cleanse the thoughts of our hearts*

by the inspiration of your Holy Spirit,
that we may perfectly love you,
and worthily magnify your holy name;
through Christ our Lord. Amen
Collect for purity

Almighty God,
whose only Son has opened for us
a new and living way into your presence:
give us pure hearts and steadfast wills
to worship you in spirit and in truth:
through Jesus your Son our Lord,
who is alive and reigns with you,
in the unity of the Holy Spirit,
one God, now and for ever. Amen
Collect for the 14th Sunday after Trinity

NINE

GRACIOUS LIVING

It is more blessed to give than to receive.[1]

A recent survey uncovered an interesting fact. Whereas under ten per cent of the population go to church on Sunday, over thirty per cent of those involved in voluntary organizations and social action groups go to church. Far from church being a place in which to hide (though that is true for some people), it is for many the place from which they draw strength and vision to serve others around them. They find that the worship of the church, the grace of God made known to them in word and sacrament, and the riches of the Judaeo-Christian heritage, sustains them in their service of others.

They are drawing strength from the living well of the Christian faith.

It is this active service that is the focus of these two Beatitudes – being merciful and pure in heart. The earlier ones have led up to this point. In being poor in spirit, the gospel calls the Christian to realize the limits of our creatureliness, and to be open to grace from God and from all of life. In mourning, we are called to be in

---

1 'In all this I have given you an example that by such work we must support the weak, remembering the words of the Lord Jesus, for he himself said, "It is more blessed to give than to receive." ' (Acts 20:35)

touch with our, and the world's, need for healing and restoration that is so evident in human lives. The Beatitudes begin with this call to 'be real', alive and open to life's joys and struggles.

Rather than urge us, in response to this awareness of life's ups and downs, to rush out and put everyone and everything right, the second pair of Beatitudes lead us to turn in faith and obedience to God. The call here is to wait for wisdom from God (meekness), and to align our hopes and desires to the central concern of God for his world: namely, righteousness.

So in living out the Beatitudes, we begin by recognizing we are creatures before the Creator. Then we are to go on to discern the will of the Creator for his creation. That is to be followed (as expressed in this third pair of Beatitudes) by action. The emphasis here is in acting with generosity towards ourselves, others and the world around us.

To engage in mission is to participate in the movement of God's love towards people, since God is a fountain of sending love.

David Bosch, *Transforming mission*

GRACIOUS LIVING

It is this that is encapsulated in the words *gracious living*. They are normally used to describe those living 'in the lap of luxury', the life of the stately home or the lifestyle of the Hollywood film star. However, does it not better describe the life of those who have discovered the grace (limitless generosity) of God and are drawing on those riches to sustain them in a lifestyle of merciful generosity and love to all whose lives they touch? They are living out what they rightly are, members of a royal family and a priestly community, caught up both in the worship of the One who is the source of mercy and in the work of divine mercy reaching into the brokenness of our world. As Peter put it:

> You are a chosen race, a royal priesthood, a holy nation, God's own people, in order that you may proclaim the mighty acts of him who called you out of darkness into his marvellous light.
>
> Once you were not a people,
> but now you are God's people;
> once you had not received mercy,
> but now you have received mercy. (1 Peter 2:9–10[2])

This focus on action characterizes the second half of the Beatitudes. We are now into the outworking of right attitudes to ourselves, life, God. As such, these two Beatitudes begin to unpack what it means not just to desire God's righteousness, but to act upon it.

In a culture where the focus is on getting, here is a call from the Christian heritage, and from the Beatitudes in particular, to order our lives around God's giving. Whereas the materialistic and consumer culture in which we live sees the aim of life as summed up in the phrase 'laughing all the way *to* the bank', the Christian is called, rather, to be part of a community which is laughing all the way *from* the bank – passing on inherited wealth to those around.

The unwritten goal of present Western culture, at the personal level, is to secure in every way possible one's material wealth and possessions. The Beatitudes open up a world shaped by awareness of resources beyond the material, and by an understanding that serving and giving are marks of what it means to live life to the

---

2 Quoting (in verse 10) Hosea 1:9–10.

full. To put it another way, Christians are as committed as the rest of our society to improving their standard of living. It is just that our 'standard of living' is measured by likeness to Christ, not least as defined by the Beatitudes.

With this in mind, we turn to explore three vital stages in this process of gracious living to which these two Beatitudes direct our steps.

LIVING OUT OF GRACE

The starting point for living graciously is to be on the receiving end of God's generosity. It is here that we notice a further parallel between the two halves of the Beatitudes. The Beatitude on mercy has close links with the first Beatitude, on being poor in spirit. When we acknowledge our human limitations, we are thereby open to the grace and mercy of God. Once we 'have received mercy' we have something out of which to live. This affects several fundamental aspects of human living.

Self-acceptance. Contrary to much popular thinking, we as Christians are not called to put self down, but rather to accept and love ourselves. The person who cannot accept themselves is unable to move out beyond the self to give attention to others; whereas the person with a healthy sense of self-worth can forget self and pay attention to the world around them. This call to begin by receiving grace, and thus with self-acceptance, is expressed in Jesus' summary of the two great commandments to love God and love others. Significantly, Jesus slips in a 'third great commandment', or rather a prior condition for obeying the other two, namely to love God and our neighbour 'as yourself'.

Christian service is not some heroic effort of putting ourselves down. It is about giving ourselves to others; and that will not happen if we feel, often at a deep instinctive level, that we are not 'a good thing' to give.

The eucharist is the basic dynamic of such gracious living, for in it we acknowledge with empty hands our need of grace and our receiving the love of God – expressed through the gift of bread and wine – and are thus equipped to 'live and work to your praise and glory'.

The apostle Paul gives us a striking image, built around baptism and the passion of Christ, for understanding the self. He speaks in several epistles about dying to self and rising with Christ, and about putting off the old nature and putting on the new nature. The call is to die to destructive ways of seeing ourselves and to say yes to God's way of seeing us. In this different approach Paul is simply giving expression to the same truth as is expressed here in the Beatitudes – that it is all done by grace. Only by receiving love can we have anything to give.

Motivation. There is a danger in seeing that all that matters is that we do 'works of mercy', yet the gospel makes it clear that the motivation matters as much as the action. It is not unknown for Christians to be motivated by guilt, ambition, or by seeking to earn acceptance from God or from others. This is why a proper discipline of confession (mourning) is needed in order that we may own the deeper motivations.

In churches in particular, there can easily be unhealthy pressure to act mercifully. Some churches engage with acts of service in order to be 'seen by men'. This is a well-intentioned desire to give a good impression. Yet Jesus specifically called the disciples to do acts of mercy simply 'before your Father in heaven'. This means that actions should arise out of a discerned sense of call. Vocation validates service – and keeps it from crushing us (Matthew 11:28–30).

What is true for churches is true for individuals too. Gracious living is freely chosen. Here again, all too easily in groups such as churches, moral pressure is put on people. 'After all,' as someone said to me recently, 'you can't say no to the vicar when he asks you to help.' My response is, and was even when I was a vicar, 'But you must!' I am not arguing for *always* saying no to the vicar, but rather always saying yes to God. Action not prompted by a response to love, ceases to partake of the nature of living by grace and so fails – even though well intentioned – to communicate that grace. This truth leads naturally to the next step.

The healthy person is someone who can live day by day and receive existence as a gift with open hands.

Jean-Jacques Suurmond, *Word and Spirit at play*

LIVING WITH GRACE

If we are to take action we need to know where we can find the tools for the job to which we have been called. They are right there in front of us in the Sermon on the Mount. There are three, for the able-bodied – prayer, giving and acts of mercy. As the years advance we may have to do just the first two, or only the first one. Yet, living on our own, even confined to our bed, that first task – prayer – can be a wonderful way to enable us to continue to be part of God's purposes in the world.

'When you pray ...' (Matthew 6:5–18). This is where the purity of heart, the vision, the courage and the energy come from. Certainly, Jesus built his whole vision, discernment and refreshment around time spent with God. Sadly in the church we find that many engaged in social action are not praying and many who are praying are not doing so for the transformation of unjust structures in our world. Yet prayer and action go hand in hand.

This prayer is not just about requests ('God bless ...'). It is about gifts of insight and wisdom; the 'seeing through' of which the sixth Beatitude speaks. We need to bring our efforts before God, and to *expect* light on the path ahead to be given to us. One of the greatest weaknesses of much prayer is that we ask, but never stay around long enough to hear the answer. Too often we put the receiver down on God. When it comes to prayer we are the receiver.

Acts of mercy and giving are assumed, not argued for, by Jesus in the Sermon on the Mount. He does not say '*if ...*', but '*when ...*'. What Jesus demonstrated in the whole of his ministry is that in doing such acts, we need continually to be co-operating with the grace of God. We do not go out on our own to serve God, but in the awareness that it is his grace which sustains and directs us. The Prayer Book Collect 'Prevent us, O Lord, in all our doings with thy most gracious favour, and further us with thy continual help' is not a request that God would stop us, but rather that he would start us! To 'prevent', as used in the Prayer Book, means to 'go before'; to prepare the ground, to be at work in the situation, to be bringing in the kingdom around, through and before us. That is what equips us to go.

I think of a mother-and-toddler group where there were no great problems. It would have been easy for the Christian leaders to take the attitude, 'Leave this one to us, God'; they had skills, experience and enthusiasm aplenty. What more could they want? Grace. It was in the willingness to pray regularly for the children, parents and families represented by those who came, that the leaders became more aware of individual needs. In part they responded simply by praying. It certainly made them more out-going towards all who came – sitting with children and parents and resisting the temptation of forming a 'leaders' clique' in the kitchen. This praying together was also what sensitized them to the needs of individuals, gave them the courage to offer to pray with or for those having various problems and, from time to time, to speak of their faith and also to extend their care beyond the times of the group meetings.

In situations like that the 'acts of mercy' are done in active co-operation with the grace of God. Those involved neither thought they could do the work without reference to God, nor did they think that 'leaving it all to God' was the way. They discovered the spiritual dynamic of collaborative working – with the grace of God.

THE TWO GREAT COMMANDMENTS

*Each demands a vulnerability, even a dying to ourselves
in the admission that we are not our own ultimate centre,
validation, or purpose.*

John F. Kavanaugh, *Still following Christ in a consumer society*

LIVING FOR GRACE

The radical nature of the way of Christ is expressed in the further Beatitude quoted by Paul that 'it is more blessed to give than to receive' (Acts 20:35). Jesus also expressed this when he said:

> Those who want to save their life will lose it, and those who lose their life for my sake will find it. For what will it profit them if they gain the whole world but forfeit their life? Or what will they give in return for their life? (Matthew 16:25–6)

This is a counter-instinctive way to live. Our instincts tell us to get, to keep, to protect and only to give if we have enough 'and to spare'. Jesus, however, lived and taught another way of life – that in giving we receive and in serving others we discover ourselves.

Such an approach brings us back to the matter of vocation explored in an earlier chapter.

It also raises for us questions about spirituality, understood from the perspective of our deepest motivation and what it is that makes sense of life. What are we living for? There are many answers to such a question. In answering it we need to distinguish between what we would like our motivation to be and what it is. They are not necessarily the same. We may be able to discern what we are living for, by paying attention to idols. Luke Johnson has the following perceptive things to say about idols:

> Idolatry, in simple terms, is the choice of treating as ultimate and absolute that which is neither absolute nor ultimate ... Functionally, then, my god is that which rivets my attention, centres my activity, preoccupies my mind, and motivates my action ... Diagnostically, I can tell what my god is by seeing what it is around which the patterns of my life organize themselves. (*Sharing possessions*, p. 49)

Positively, we can discern how we are to work with and for the grace of God by paying attention to vocation. Doing so protects us from becoming overstretched and at the mercy of pressure from endless and unrealistic demands. To give ourselves freely we need to develop an ability to know the limits of our strength and an ability to set limits. There can be no authentic yes to serving others unless we have developed the skill and courage to say no. We often find that difficult and then express it in terms of 'What will people think of me?' That very response suggests that we have not yet let God's call be our overriding concern and vision; nor that we have yet reached the ability to trust our reputation to God.

Giving ourselves to gracious living quickly reminds us that we have limited resources. It is vital that we avoid playing God or thinking we can save the world. We cannot, but we can play our part. And our part is just that – a part. So our need is to discern what that part is.

Not least is this necessary today because the media in general, and TV in particular, bombard us with the most desperate needs as they emerge, every day, from across the globe. We cannot solve, or even help in, all these situations. What we can do all too easily, however, is to use the overwhelming nature of the problems as an excuse to do nothing. Rather it should prompt us to find something we can do and get on and do it. We can give thanks for that calling, pray for mercy and vision (purity of heart), for us in our work and for others engaged in other projects, and let God retain ultimate responsibility for His world. So choosing a specific project, focus, task, concern is the way to ensure we join in without going under.

JUBILEE ACTIONS

One of the great themes of the Old Testament which lay behind the ministry of Jesus is that of jubilee. It was really an extension of sabbath, with particular emphasis on being directed outwards to others. The sabbath principle, of a rest every seven days, was extended into the sabbath year of rest for the land when crops were not sown on land that had been cultivated for the past six years. By extension this was then given focus in the year of jubilee, which was the fiftieth year – after seven series of sabbath years.

In that fiftieth year, slaves were set free, debts were cancelled, land was rested, property (including land) was returned to its owner and a great party was had by all. This was the vision that inspired Jesus' whole ministry, as is seen in his first sermon:

When he came to Nazareth, where he had been brought up, he went to the synagogue on the sabbath day, as was his custom. He stood up to read, and the scroll of the prophet Isaiah was given to him. He unrolled the scroll and found the place where it was written:

'The Spirit of the Lord is upon me,

because he has anointed me
>to bring good news to the poor.

He has sent me to proclaim release to captives
>and recovery of sight to the blind,
>>to let the oppressed go free,

to proclaim the year of the Lord's favour.'

... Then he began to say to them, 'Today this scripture is fulfilled in your hearing.' (Luke 4:16–21)

Jesus, in the Beatitudes, pronounces God's blessing on those who will share with him in this gracious work of setting captives free, giving hope to the hopeless and help to those amongst whom we live.

It certainly involves specific acts of mercy and service – something that is a fundamental part of what it means to follow Christ. 'Hands on' service of others is a core curriculum subject for disciples. That service includes the caring support of others with whom we live, work and worship. It also reaches to the farthest corners of the earth.

One particular way in which this gracious living, and the theme of jubilee, is currently being expressed is by the Jubilee 2000 campaign for the cancelling of the debts of some of the poorest nations of the world. It is a good reminder that we do not have to resign ourselves to powerlessness in the face of seemingly insuperable problems. We can, as the saying goes, light a candle rather than curse the darkness. We can add our voice, our efforts, to that of many others and find that power is given to move mountains.[3]

---

3 Details about the Jubilee 2000 campaign, including copies of their workbook for groups, *The Debt cutters handbook*, can be obtained from Jubilee 2000, PO Box 100, London SE1 7RT.

*Our aim is to celebrate the millennium by lifting
the burden of unpayable debt from the poorest countries.*

Debt cutters handbook

JUBILEE ATTITUDES

Jubilee is also a challenge to us about our motivation in relationships with those whom we live and work with. What is our goal in these relationships? It is quite legitimate to ask what we are hoping to get from such relationships. As those who are poor in spirit, we need to be open to the grace of God as it comes to us through other people. But also, it is imperative that we ask what is it that God is calling us to give to these people, what are we called to contribute to these relationships, what is it that God is calling us to contribute to creating in these settings? In other words, gracious living is not only engagement in *acts of service*, it is also about an *attitude of service*. Indeed the acts grow out of the attitudes.

This attitude of service is itself to be marked, as jubilee indicates, not by a sense of servile drudgery and duty, but by inviting others to join in with the celebration of God's goodness and life's richness. Gracious living is a freely chosen and joyfully expressed attitude of loving service to those we live and work with, and a compassionate care for all who share in God's creation.

PART FOUR:
Living differently

Peacemaking does not mean

◆ keeping everybody happy – it is about making (creating) something

◆ pretending wrong does not matter. It is not good to ignore conflict in the home, church or world. Nor is it usually advisable or holy to pretend wrong is not happening

◆ ending hostilities – truce-making may be a vital first step but peacemaking is more.

Rather it is about ...

◆ taking part in God's mission – to bring everything into harmony/balance/wholeness.

◆ practical expression of respect for all people and all of creation. It includes peacemaking in families, communities, nations and the environment, and the just and joyful distribution of the world's resources.

TEN

THE WHOLE STORY

Blessed are the peacemakers,
for they will be called children of God.

There is more to peacemaking than keeping people happy. Not that 'turning a blind eye' or 'pouring oil on troubled waters' is to be despised. Without them our marriages, homes, churches and places of work would be the worse. Little acts of kindness, anticipating and then finding the way around potential 'flashpoints', and simply smiling can all make life more peaceful to all concerned. We take these little steps almost instinctively. They are like a good diet – they prevent more serious illnesses later on.

Sometimes, however, our ailments need more than a good diet. They need medicine. So too the ailments of the human heart and of human society. The sickness and brokenness can only be relieved by a good dose of repentance and forgiveness, together with what doctors now call 'a different regime'. Facing and dealing with the barriers to peace is essential repair work on the fabric of our relationships. Yet how hard we find it to 'take in' our own forgiveness, let alone find any spare to give to others who have crossed our path or our plans. And how hard we find it to adjust to those regimes; to different responses and changed perspectives which are needed to avoid the old ailments.

There is more radical work needed as well. It is a work that addresses deep-seated pain and lack of peace. We see the need for it in the breakdown of families, the fragmentation of communities and the seemingly intractable conflicts at the global level made all too obvious in places such as Bosnia, the Middle East and Northern Ireland.

This deeper work is about addressing root causes and finding ways of bringing about change. The image of the good diet or the necessary medicine gives way to the picture of the surgeon's knife. Wielded with skill, dedication and delicacy, it is none the less a disturbing and painful action. It is done to cut out the destructive forces and to give the body's natural healing instincts a chance to gain the upper hand.

I heard recently of how some healthy cells in the body attack cancerous cells. When they come across them, they pull back, form themselves into a torpedo shape and hurl themselves at the destructive cell. With considerable force they penetrate the shell of the harmful cell and then 'explode on impact', destroying both themselves and the cancer. It is amazing that our bodies can do all this without even letting us know! It is a picture at the biological level of the costs involved in sustaining or achieving wholeness. It is also a fascinating illustration of how like warfare peacemaking can be.

From the cancerous body, through the dysfunctional family and the church in conflict, to the body politic, we stand urgently in need of peacemaking understood as a health-giving dynamic. To this end we have a double need; both to understand the richness and scope of what peace is, and also to find help in discovering what part we can play to bring it about.

THE PEACE OF THE LORD

When we turn to Christ's life and work it seems as if everything he did was about peacemaking. Healing, teaching, confronting, dying and rising are all aspects of the work of making peace. It is helpful to see the various levels on which this peacemaking was conducted.

Healing the body. This is the most evident and visible aspect of Jesus' work of bringing peace to individuals. Touching the leper, restoring the crippled, the blind and the deaf are central aspects of Christ's ministry.

The development of hospitals and our modern understanding of sickness and healing have been enormously stimulated by Christ's impact on Western culture. The recovery of the healing ministry in the church, despite its limitations and the occasional extravagant claims made on its behalf, is part of the peacemaking work of Christ through today's church.

This care for the physical condition and circumstances of others has inspired, in recent decades, fresh expressions of concern for those deprived of the necessities of life. Oxfam, Christian Aid, CAFOD, Tear Fund, Jubilee 2000 and many other groups are seeking to express today this peacemaking work of care for people's physical circumstances. They express the passion for justice in terms of a more equitable distribution of the world's riches, for peacemaking includes the just and generous sharing of resources.

Each year the Third World pays the West three times more in debt repayments than it receives in aid.

Debt cutters handbook

However, healing is needed not only in the physical realm. The development of disciplines such as psychiatry, and the emergence of alternative medicine and of counselling services, all point to the fact that healing is a multi-faceted process.

The cure of souls. This is the older term for the work of counselling and spiritual direction. It reminds us that Jesus' concern for people did not stop at the level of physical need. In the gospel stories we frequently see Jesus addressing not just physical symptoms, but factors such as forgiveness, self-acceptance, faith and hope which are also needed for full health. This aspect of healing, and of peacemaking, reminds us that peace very often begins in the mind and in our attitude to ourselves and the world around us.

Central to the work of peacemaking is bringing people into right relationship with God. Once that process begins it leads on to, and finds expression in, the putting right of other relationships. We see this process of evangelism-leading-to-a-changed-lifestyle again and again in Jesus' engagement with individuals. Saying to the paralytic, 'Your sins are forgiven you,' to the Samaritan woman, 'Go and fetch your husband,' to Zacchaeus, 'I must come to your house today,' and to Bartimaeus, 'What do you want me to do for you?' are all part of this peacemaking process. They provoked those whom he addressed to 'see' a different future.

Peace begins in the mind, with our attitude to God, life, others and – crucially – to ourselves too. It is where peacemaking flows out of purity of heart. We need to 'see' the future if we are to enter into it. This is what is meant by bringing hope into a situation – it is giving people the vision of a new and better future.

Spiritual direction, counselling, the healing power of a listening ear and the work of community building are all ways in which we see this at work today. We see it too in the communities of reconciliation in Northern Ireland, and the work of contemporary expressions of Christian action such as Samaritans and the Hospice movement.

Hospitality. Jesus saw a strong social dimension to the work of healing. He was continually 'going out of his way' to count others in. Touching the leper, partying with the prostitutes and tax collectors, befriending the soldiers of the occupying forces, were all forms of social healing. Jesus minded the gap between different groups who feared each other and wrote each other off, and stepped out across all divides to bring shalom, harmony, peace.

Simple acts of welcome, and listening to the stories of other people, can help here. They enable us to feel the exclusion others feel and to understand their actions too. This aspect of peacemaking can be seen in the work of women's refuges, in work amongst asylum seekers, in the care and support of those released from prison, and efforts to communicate with and gain the confidence of travellers and the gypsy community. It is manifest also wherever we reach out to newcomers to our churches, whether from the local community or from other countries.

In a divided and often suspicious culture, peacemakers are those who reach out, physically to touch, and to give hospitality. Hospitality is not just about inviting people into our homes. It is about communities being 'open spaces' where the newcomer is welcomed. Counting others in rarely happens without our putting ourselves out.

Confronting injustice. It is impossible, in reading the gospels, to miss the disturbing nature of Jesus' ministry, well expressed in those words of his which seem to contradict this Beatitude, namely:

> Do you think that I have come to bring peace to the earth? No, I tell you, but rather division! (Luke 12:51)

How far removed that is from notions of 'gentle Jesus meek and mild'. We see him living out this truth when he speaks of Herod as 'that fox', challenges the scribes and Pharisees, warns of the dangers of hypocrisy, confronts the disciples' 'lust for power', casts out demons and overturns the tables of the money-changers in the Temple. None of these actions fits easily into our stained-glass image of Jesus as a man who would never disturb anyone. The truth is that he was a powerful and uncomfortable presence on the edge of society, whom the powers-that-be continually felt threatened by. These disturbing actions are akin to the surgeon's knife; seemingly acting against his settled purpose yet actually carrying forward the ultimate goal – of wholeness.

To share today in Christ's peacemaking work involves us in the same range of activities; caring about people's bodies and physical well-being, addressing underlying negative and hostile attitudes that block wholeness and justice, engaging in radical actions of counting others in rather than keeping them out, and being prepared for the deep conflicts that are required if we are to 'give peace a chance'.

DISTURBING THE UN-PEACE

It is at just this point that we want to walk quietly away and avoid getting involved. Peacemaking as confronting injustice, uncovering destructive motives, cutting out cancerous growths in communities and in organizations, facing the power struggles that occur wherever human beings come together, seems like dangerous work. It is.

Is it not better and wiser to 'let sleeping dogs lie'? If everyone is happy with the present situation, what is to be gained by uncovering these things? The answer is that not everyone is happy. Unjust structures always favour the insiders and rob others, usually the powerless and often the majority, of their place in the whole enterprise.

Seeing that this is so is a vital first step in peacemaking. Without a vision of a better future and a better way there can be no challenge to what is, which is why the 'seeing' involved in being pure of heart is the essential preparation for peacemaking. We need to see what could be.

But there is a cost, and it is the cost of disturbing the *status quo*. Jesus, in confronting the religious and political leaders, certainly got himself into a great deal of trouble. It cost him his life. So it did for Martin Luther King, when he sought to address the un-peace of racial segregation. Christians in South Africa and in East Germany were instrumental, in their different ways, in the overthrow of unjust regimes. They frequently found themselves hounded by the authorities, who did not want the un-peace disturbing.

Wilberforce and Shaftesbury devoted much of their lives to the cause of the abolition of slavery, fighting costly personal battles against 'vested interests'. Peacemakers are often seen simply as troublemakers.

It is this work of peacemaking that is central to Christ's going 'the way of the cross'. He was confronting the unjust structures of the occupying army and the colluding religious establishment. He was also addressing the unjust hearts of the people who were so ready to be manipulated into calling for his death, the weakness of the disciples in making themselves scarce, betraying and denying him, and the willingness of everyone to settle for less than God's purposes for the city and its people. All of these destructive elements are brought to the light and healed through a love that bears the pain of their corrosive acids rather than paying back 'in kind'.

It is this vision that strengthens Jesus' arm to disturb the un-peace – the uneasy truce, compromise, injustice and exclusion which characterized the city over which he had wept.

THE FAMILY BUSINESS

The work of peace is at the heart of the whole mission of Christ – gathering up all creation into the loving purposes of God. That is why the promise is that those who choose this way, rather than opting for apathy or hostility, will be called children of God. They are involving themselves in the family business. Those who engage in the work of reconciliation between groups and individuals, those who work to bring people to a right relationship with God, and those who seek to confront injustice, are risk takers after the heart of God – who put himself out to make peace with humanity. Some of the steps that we can take are as follows.

Facing reality and getting others to do so. Often the biggest task is to get people to look problems in the face. Sometimes ingenious ways need to be found to get people to see that something should be done, that a problem needs addressing. Typically this is often the real obstacle to true peace in our marriages. Facing our part in the problems that confront us is the biggest obstacle to peace. In organizations the same problem exists; getting those with the power to bring about change to face the changes that are needed. Often their power and control will be one of the things that needs to be 'renegotiated'.

Getting people to talk. What a marvellous healing this can be, but it is a skill not only getting the reticent to talk, but also helping the confident and vocal to listen. There are skills here that can be learned, but simply getting people and groups to talk with the aid of a 'referee' can bring about change. In leading training days for churches during my present work I sometimes think that getting church members, clergy and laity, to sit down and talk to each other is the single most important part of the day. Equally, in the work of communicating the Christian faith, my experience has often been that praying with people is better than arguing with them. Talking to God definitely has the edge on talking about God.

Looking for a 'win-win' solution. Inevitably, in the early stages the 'warring parties' are looking simply to win, not least by ensuring that the 'other party' loses. Reconciliation happens, and injustice is addressed, when they can share a common hope about the future and invest something of themselves in helping the other party to achieve their goals and hopes.

I recall being involved in counselling a couple whose marriage seemed close to collapse. They had spent the evening telling each other, with me acting as referee, all that was wrong with the marriage. In this they were agreed – that the problem was 'you'! It had been necessary work to bring this negative and critical material to the surface, otherwise it could never be owned and dealt with. Wondering what we had achieved and where we could go next, I felt prompted to say, 'Having listened to your partner, is there one thing you could offer to put into the relationship, which would be of help to them?' They both became silent at this point. Then he made a simple offer of practical help. She responded by offering to listen more sensitively in future. Several further 'gifts' followed. The destructive dynamic was broken. I left them in each other's arms! I hasten to add that it was an exception to my normal experience in marriage conflicts; but it was a wonderful experience of seeing people start to work for the good of the other – building *shalom*, becoming peacemakers.

Looking beyond the local. There is so much lack of peace in the immediate world to which we relate that it is easy to forget the global village of which we are part. Yet the plight of the powerless, the starving, oppressed and fearful cries out for our attention. We cannot save the world, but we can join in at some point in this global vision. We do need to raise our vision beyond the immediate and local, for those very situations need the bigger vision and the perspective of these global needs. The Christian faith encourages us not to be daunted, but to be part of an army of people expressing God's loving concern for his whole created order.

All shall be included in the Feast of life
Christian Aid 50th anniversary statement, 1995

THE FAMILY LIKENESS

The striking promise in this Beatitude is that those who make peace will be called children of God. It underlines just how central to the nature of God peacemaking is. It is how righteousness works out in a fallen world; not in judgement and condemnation but in bringing the fragments together, and building a new picture and experience of harmony.

This is a profoundly reassuring promise. It tells us that God invests himself in such work. Costly, risky and painful though peacemaking is, God gives himself – by putting his nature, the blessing of his family likeness, into those engaged in such work. We are not on our own. God promises not only to be with us, but in us.

This work is also, in fact, instinctive in the human heart. Most of us, for example, when we hear that a marriage is 'on the rocks' would love to be able to step in and bring people back together again. We talk, when we hear of situations of conflict, about 'knocking some heads together'; but actually our instincts are usually better than that. Our desire is to join hearts as one, rather than knock heads together. The urge to find the way through to harmony, balance and joy is deep in all of us. The disciple is to expect this instinct to be activated by the indwelling of Christ, by the Spirit.

Our calling is to be sensitive to that instinct, alive to the prompting of the Spirit, and willing to take the risky action which that instinct and prompting make us aware of. When we do so, we tap into the very nature of God. That is an bottomless reservoir of grace that can bring hope to the most hopeless of situations. It is also an amazing promise that when we do engage in peacemaking, something of the very character of God rubs off on us.

Meditation

Blessed are the peacemakers, for they will be called the children of God.

We come before you that we may serve your peace-creating purposes
We rejoice to share in the Christ-like work of bringing all things to a good End

READINGS

Seek the welfare of the city where I have sent you into exile, and pray to the Lord on its behalf, for in its welfare you will find your welfare.

(Jeremiah 29:7)

[Abraham] looked forward to a city that has foundations, whose architect and builder is God.

(Hebrews 11:10)

How very good and pleasant it is
when kindred live together in unity!
It is like the precious oil on the head,
running down upon the beard,
on the beard of Aaron, running down
over the collar of his robes.

It is like the dew of Hermon,
  which falls on the mountains of Zion.
For there the Lord ordained his blessing,
  life for evermore.
(Psalm 133)

HYMNS

He shall come down like showers
  Upon the fruitful earth,
And love, joy, hope, like flowers,
  Spring in his path to birth:
Before him on the mountains
  Shall peace, the herald, go;
And righteousness in fountains
  From hill to valley flow.
James Montgomery

Lord, your summons echoes true
when you but call my name.
Let me turn and follow you
and never be the same.
In your company I'll go
where your love and footsteps show.
Thus I'll move and live and grow
in you, and you in me.
John L. Bell and Graham Maule

REFLECTION

What city (or group of people) has God called us to live among and to
  serve?

- *what would peace*, shalom, *look like in this setting?*
- *what steps can we take to help move in this direction?*
- *what obstacles need to be removed (in us, and others, in the ethos of the group)?*

Blessed are the peacemakers, for they will be called the children of God.

PRAYERS

Almighty Father,
whose will is to restore all things
in your beloved Son, the king of all:
govern the hearts and minds of those in authority,
and bring the families of the nations,
divided and torn apart by the ravages of sin,
to be subject to his just and gentle rule
who is alive and reigns with you,
in the unity of the Holy Spirit,
one God, now and for ever. Amen
Collect for the 3rd Sunday before Advent

Lord, make us instruments of your peace.
Where there is hatred, let us sow love;
where there is injury, pardon;
where there is discord, union;
where there is doubt, faith;
where there is despair, hope;
where there is darkness, light; where there is sadness, joy;
for your mercy and your truth's sake. Amen
The prayer of St Francis

Persecution does not mean

- being insensitive – and not caring about the impact of what we say and do
- that Christians should be 'looking for trouble' (persecution comes from being peacemakers, being shot at from both sides)
- that we have a mandate to fight with everyone who disagrees with us.

Rather it is about ...

- standing out from the crowd. We are to be willing to be thought odd and/or subversive; or politely sidelined or ignored
- speaking and standing up for what is true and right – whatever the response
- accepting the consequences of living by different values.

ELEVEN

THE COST OF LIVING

Blessed are those who are persecuted for righteousness' sake,
for theirs is the kingdom of heaven.

Persecution is an embarrassment to Western Christians; or rather, the lack of it is. There is so much in the scriptures that prepares the disciple for a rough ride, for suffering and pain, in this world that when it does not happen we are thrown by the experience. Are we simply not worth persecuting, we wonder? Not that most normal people are looking for it. It is just that there is an underground stream of dis-ease, even guilt, about the lack of it.

This is not to suggest that Christians never have life made difficult for them. From time to time it does happen. Some resign over a matter of conscience, some are ostracized in little ways that irritate rather than threaten. For a good number, 'persecution' (and they would be reluctant to use such a grandiose concept to describe their experience) takes the form of jokes about language and sexual innuendos with comments such as, 'Sorry, I forgot the holy man was here', 'Pardon me, saint Jane,' and 'Sorry, I forgot you were the religious one.' Sir Cliff Richard's comment – 'I would rather be laughed at than thrown to the lions' – sums up the normal level of persecution for many in the West, and the right attitude to what we do experience.

However, some followers of Christ within today's 'anything goes' Western culture do experience real persecution, simply because they insist that not everything does 'go'. It may come in the form of sexual harrassment as an expression of the need to gain power (either as 'conquest' or 'seduction') over another. For others it comes when a stand is made about dishonesty to clients or customers. Some are pressurized about working all hours, not least Sundays. Yet others are accused of being unreal, disloyal or disruptive if they will not conform to a corrupt, immoral or dishonest culture. These are very real pressures which the church rarely speaks of. Certainly much less is heard of these things from the pulpit compared with the amount experienced by church members in daily living. Nothing that follows should be seen as belittling the real experience of such 'persecution' in the lives of many Christians in the 'civilised West'. The young, starting out in work situations, are particularly vulnerable to this sort of pressure. They need the understanding and support of fellow Christians and their churches. These issues are not matters to be swept under the carpet, but rather to be brought into the light of Christ.

Before exploring the issue of persecution today we need to think first about its nature as portrayed in the New Testament.

THE FIGHT OF FAITH

The New Testament has three categories of difficulties that the disciple is likely to face.

The first is temptation: being drawn away from what is right. This was the very first experience of 'opposition' that Jesus encountered when, immediately after his baptism, he was led by the Spirit into the wilderness to be tempted. The passage is so familiar we lose some of its striking nature. Having just seen Jesus affirmed as the beloved Son of God, and having had that confirmed by the descent of the Spirit in the form of a dove, it makes strange reading to see the next work of the Spirit was to 'lead him into temptation'. Yet temptation is the inevitable consequence of a 'choice culture', indeed a 'choice universe' such as God has established. We can only love if we are free not to love. Love cannot be coerced. It has to be a freely chosen response. The strengthening of holy responses comes through testing, of which the first stage is temptation. Just as gold needs fire to purify it, and as plants need gravity to 'grow against',[1] so human beings need true and false choices if they are ever to choose love freely. It is friends and family who are the channels of this pressure on Jesus. Seduction is the keynote of temptation.

The second is testing or trial: being pushed off the right way. This is the persecution stage. It is the pressure to quit and opt for the quiet and comfortable life. It was what provoked the disciples to run away when Jesus most needed them – at his death. It was what caused Peter to deny Jesus: the pressure to keep his distance was too great. Oppression and fear are the forces behind trial and persecution. In the life of Jesus it is the scribes and Pharisees (representatives of the religious structures) who spearhead this pressure on Jesus, culminating in the calling in of Rome to help them destroy him.

The third is tribulation: the inescapable upheaval of the End Times. The book of Revelation is full of vivid imagery of the trials that will be bound up with the final coming of Christ. Babylon, the great harlot, is the central image: it is one of a city bent on afflicting and destroying God's people. The new Jerusalem (notice it is a holy city,

---

1   See the chapter 'Sin – the gravity of our situation' in my book *Being human, being church* for a fuller exploration of these issues.

not a return to the idyllic garden metaphor of Eden) is the city that finally emerges, but not before much suffering on the part of God's chosen ones.

There is always the temptation in us to settle for the easy way.

Kathy Galloway, *Struggles to love*

JESUS AS SUFFERING SERVANT

It is in the life of Christ that we see all three of these elements at work. His ministry begins with the forty-day fast in the wilderness in which he is tempted by the devil. What is happening here is that he is being enticed to conform to expectations, surrendering the inner loyalty to God in the process.

The story of his ministry is one of growing hostility from the religious leaders. It begins with difficult questions, goes on to hostile accusations and character assassinations, and ends in the lynch mob of the cross. The build-up seems inexorable.

In his death, Christ shapes the template of all suffering, including that of the End Times. Indeed his death is the prefiguring of the End in which life triumphs in and through death, love expresses itself most fully in the context of hatred and rejection, and God is found to be Lord over all in the midst of this turmoil. As Isaiah put it, he was a man of sorrow 'despised and rejected by others', and yet 'out of his anguish he shall see light' (Isaiah 53:3, 11).

In all this there is no evidence of Jesus looking for or courting trouble. Rather, he set his face to discover and do the will of God, come what may. It was that steadfast following of his deepest vocation that led him into trouble – and through into triumph.

The goal is not persecution, but holding on to the will of God. The Beatitude alerts us to the fact that there may well be a real cost in following our vocation, but that problems and trials should neither come as a surprise nor knock us off our guard. We know that, in following Christ, we will be sustained and that any suffering will bear fruit in the long run. For us, as it was for Jesus, trials are the consequence of being fully alive to God and to the world around us. As we seek to join in with what we see the Father doing, there will be times when we discover the real cost of living. Living, that is, a life pleasing to the Father.

Jesus was put to death because he put his preaching into practice.

Michael Crosby, *Spirituality of the Beatitudes*

PERSECUTION IN CONTEXT

The setting of the church in the New Testament, and the experience of much of the church down the history of the Christian era and across the globe, is that of living in an overtly hostile culture where being known as a Christian is, if not actually life-threatening, then at least a real and distinct disadvantage as far as security, status and employment are concerned.

The church in the West is in a different and relatively unusual setting. A number of things make this setting different.

We are part of a Christian culture. However far we might think that Western civilization has strayed from its Christian roots, it remains none the less a fact that Christianity is the tradition in which the culture has been nurtured. That certainly makes persecution where most people experience it – from the state – an unlikely eventuality. The change is well expressed by two interesting facts at the time of the establishing of Christendom, under Constantine. In AD 323 it was illegal for those who owned allegiance to Christ to be in the army. They were considered dangerous and always liable to be subversive – why else would they not offer sacrifices to the emperor? In AD 423, it was impossible to be in the army if you were *not* a Christian! They were the only ones whom the state saw as having a proven loyalty to the emperor. How quickly and totally the wheels of history turned.

It is unlikely that the state, in a Christendom culture, would engage in persecuting Christians. Not least is this so because persecution is usually of a minority by the majority culture. (We have seen that demonizing of a minority at its most graphic and gruesome in the persecution of Jews during the Second World War.) The arm of the state most frequently engaging in persecution is the army, or in contemporary culture, the police force. There are certainly instances of such persecution, but they are, true to type, the persecution of minorities (ethnic and social groupings such as gypsies and homosexuals).

What Christians have to guard against, when they form the dominant culture in any setting, is that they are more likely to be perpetrators of persecution rather than its victims. The doctrine (note the word) of apartheid in South Africa is a classic case of this.

Seduction not oppression is our problem. When, as in the days of Nero, the church was fiercely persecuted, it was easy to know who the enemy was and where the threat might come from. But in our culture the nature of the 'lie' under which we live is not the oppressive or hostile powers-that-be, but the seductive 'lie' of the market. When oppression rules, as for the children of Israel in Egypt before the exodus, or for Christians in the former communist lands, everyone knows the destructive nature of the regime and longs for freedom. When materialism is the governing theme, then we are not wanting to flee from it (or, at least, most are not), but rather are eager to have 'a slice of the cake'. The culture then becomes seductive. That is the case today for the church in the West. It is actually a more dangerous state than outright oppression; but it does not feel like it. It simply feels 'comfortable'.

Apathy is the nature of the surrounding culture. Apathy is a mark of our culture. Boredom and being 'not bothered' are endemic. If that is the case, persecution is unlikely to happen – or rather the hostile force which the believer faces is *indifference* rather than *hostility*. It is certainly more comfortable that way. But apathy is very debilitating. Getting no response to costly sacrifices undermines the cost of the effort. It also indicates where our culture may want to put pressure on believers – wherever we show *passion*; for apathy means literally 'absence of passion'.

When anything goes little gets objected to. Western Christians live in a culture that has removed many of the constraints of social respectability. Much of that is good. No longer is the girl who becomes pregnant whisked away out of the community and put in an institution under a moralizing and harsh regime. Now 'anything goes', which means that there is little or no response to anyone's choice of lifestyle, whether it be focused around the worship of Christ, the pursuit of power or addiction to shopping.

All these factors add up to the real problem of getting any response, whether positive or negative, to a moral stand or a testimony of faith. 'If that's what turns you on ...' is the response we may well meet.

We do well to recognize that getting little or no response has a long-term debilitating effect. It is a subtle form of pressure to be 'not bothered'. Its power is in the very weakness of the response it gives. The weakness of response suggests that what was done in the first place was weak and not worth responding to. Acceptance of any and every lifestyle, creed and viewpoint can sap the energy out of the strongest of convictions. It certainly does not make costly choices easy. It hardly seems worth the effort.

We do not become prophets simply because
we go around being rude to and about everybody else.

Simon Tugwell, *The Beatitudes*

MARGINAL PERSECUTION

The point has already been made that it is those on the margins of society who tend to get persecuted, not the 'conforming' majority. However, we need to recognize the forces at work in our culture which are marginalizing faith. Privatizing is a way of permitting something to exist but not as foundational to 'public life'. In many ways our culture has marginalized values ('anything goes', only value what 'works' and can be counted). So, for example, it is quite acceptable in our culture for a counsellor to let their psychological studies affect their faith, but quite 'unprofessional' to allow their faith to affect the way they conduct their counselling.

A major form of persecution – far removed from being thrown to the lions – which the church faces today is this dynamic of being pushed to the margins. The Orthodox theologian Alexander Schmemann has put it, in the American context, in these words (the same process is at work in other parts of the Western world):

An American 'secularist' may be a very 'religious' man, attached to his Church, regular in attending services, generous in his contributions, punctual in prayer. But all this does not in the least alter the plain fact that his understanding of all these aspects of his life –

154

marriage, family, home and profession, and ultimately his religious obligations themselves – is derived not from the creed he confesses in Church ... but from 'philosophies of life', that is, ideas and convictions having virtually nothing to do with that creed, if not directly opposed to it. One has only to enumerate some of the key 'values' of our culture – success, status, security, competition, profit, prestige, ambition – to realize that they are at the opposite pole from the entire *ethos* and inspiration of the Gospel ...
Alexander Schmemann, *Great Lent*,
St Vladimir's Seminary Press, 1974, p. 108

It may well be that in standing against this marginalizing of faith that the Christian will discover that persecution – not least of the 'laughed at' variety – is quickly awakened. Really to allow the values, as spelt out in the Beatitudes and explored here, to shape our lifestyle, will certainly challenge the assumed perspective of the consumer culture.

The calling of the church, at this point, may be to heed the voices of people like Bishop Lesslie Newbigin who called the church to face this marginalizing, and to find ways of moving out beyond such limitations. A church committed to the comfortable life is unlikely to be willing to make such a journey. A church seeking to live by the Beatitudes will find themselves already well down a path through life that passes through the territory of persecution, however subtle the form.

THE COST OF LIVING

When Jesus called Bartimaeus forward he asked him a simple, yet shocking question, 'What do you want me to do?' If ever a person was put on the spot ...! Bartimaeus seems to have had no hesitation. Of course his need was obvious. But he risked all in daring to ask for nothing less than the impossible – and his faith was rewarded. He saw and his whole life was transformed. He was made whole and restored not just to full health but to full participation in society; its joys, freedom, opportunities and its responsibilities. Many doors were now open to him, but no doubt it all felt strange, disturbing and uncomfortable – as well as overwhelmingly wonderful.

We, individually, as a church and in the whole of our society need the same healing today. We need to see. We need a fresh vision of what could be. Like Bartimaeus, however, we may find that really being alive to God's purposes involves some costly and disturbing experiences.

The twentieth century opened, certainly in the Western world, on a note of great optimism. *Progress* was the key word. It ends in something more like cynicism – the absence of hope. In the church, all too easily, our eyes are on the past; whether the good old days when more people went to church, or further back on the riches of our Christian heritage. Our sights need to be set on what will be: on a vision of the purposes of God being worked out in our world today. Only when the future calls us forward can we expect to give hope to a culture which is at one and the same time both cynical and searching. It is in having a hope worth not only dying for, but living for, that Christians can fulfil their calling today.

Paul, in a striking passage in Romans, reflects on the relationship between vision and suffering from an illuminating angle. In doing so he shows what is involved when we seek to participate in what someone has described as 'God's love affair with all creation'. He writes:

I consider that the sufferings of this present time are not worth comparing with the glory about to be revealed to us. For the creation waits with eager longing for the revealing of the children of God; for the creation was subjected to futility, not of its own will but by the will of the one who subjected it, in hope that the creation itself will be set free from its bondage to decay and will obtain the freedom of the glory of the children of God. We know that the whole creation has been groaning in labour pains until now; and not only the creation, but we ourselves, who have the first fruits of the Spirit, groan inwardly while we wait for adoption, the redemption of our bodies. For in hope we were saved. Now hope that is seen is not hope. For who hopes for what is seen: But if we hope for what we do not see, we wait for it with patience.

Likewise the Spirit helps us in our weakness; for we do not know how to pray as we ought, but that very Spirit intercedes with sighs too deep for words. And God, who searches the heart, knows what is the mind of the Spirit, because the Spirit intercedes for the saints according to the will of God. (Romans 8:18–27)

The repeated refrain is that of *groaning*; referred to in three contexts. The groaning of creation as it awaits its liberation. The groaning of the believer who 'waits for our adoption', the fulfilment of redemption at the end of time. And the groaning of the Spirit who prays with 'sighs too deep for words' within us.

This puts our struggles into a bigger context. We are part of that mission of God, initiated in Christ, which has addressed the struggles of the whole creation. It involves the conversion, indeed transformation, of the individual, it involves the whole of human society with all its broken and dysfunctional structures and injustices, and it includes the whole created order too. We are part of a bigger venture and need to see all creation sharing in our struggles to come to the fullness that God has planned for us and it – together. Moreover, God is involved in this struggle too, for by His Spirit He is praying in and through us.

Indeed this work of the Spirit 'brooding' over the believer is all of a piece with the other great 'brooding' works of the Spirit: creation (Genesis 1:2) and the birth of Christ (Luke 1:35). This puts our struggles in context. We are caught up in the ongoing work of the Spirit in bringing God's purposes to their fulfilment.

The word for groaning is travail. These are labour pains, for they herald the delivery of something new. What is being brought to birth is the new creation about which Paul writes. Such an image puts our struggles and difficult times in an altogether more positive light. They do not ultimately happen just because the world is so far from God, but because they are the labour pains of this new order of reality which is the long-term goal of the kingdom.

No wonder the promise for those who suffer persecution is that 'theirs is the kingdom of heaven'.

This final Beatitude is then a call to hold on to this bigger vision of the kingdom, a challenge to resist the temptations and pressures to settle for less and for the comfortable life, and a promise that in being faithful to God's kingdom we will discover what living is really all about. It is, in the final issue, a call to engage with God our Father in his work of 'bringing all things to a good End'.

THE KINGDOM

... is about the ability to engage, contemplatively and creatively,
in the right relationships that will beget a new world order,
characterized by justice, love, peace and liberation for all.

Diarmuid O'Murchu, *Reclaiming spirituality*

Meditation

Blessed are those who are persecuted for righteousness' sake,
for theirs is the kingdom of heaven.
We come before you knowing that testing is involved in walking your way
We rejoice that, by your power, love will conquer all

READINGS

You are the salt of the earth: but if the salt has lost its taste, how can its saltiness be restored? It is no longer good for anything, but is thrown out and trampled under foot. You are the light of the world. A city built on a hill cannot be hid. No one after lighting a lamp puts it under the bushel basket, but on the lampstand, and it gives light to all in the house. In the same way, let your light shine before others, so that they may see your good works and give glory to your Father in heaven.

(Matthew 5:13–16)

The Lord has given me
the tongue of a teacher
that I may know how to sustain
the weary with a word.
Morning by morning he wakens –
wakens my ear
to listen as those who are taught.
The Lord God has opened my ear,
and I was not rebellious,
I did not turn backward.
I gave my back to those who struck me,
and my cheeks to those who pulled
out the beard;
I did not hide my face
from insult and spitting.

(Isaiah 50:4–6)

HYMNS

Father, hear the prayer we offer
Not for ease that prayer shall be
But for strength that we may ever
Live our lives courageously.

Not for ever in green pastures
Do we ask our way to be
But the steep and rugged pathway
May we tread rejoicingly.
Love Maria Willis

Whoso beset him round
    with dismal stories,
Do but themselves confound;
    His strength the more is.
No lion can him fright;
    He'll with a giant fight,
But he will have the right
    To be a pilgrim.
Percy Dearmer, after John Bunyan

REFLECTION

> *What are the marks and values of the Beatitude that God is calling us*
> *to exhibit?*
>
> *Where do pressures to conform inhibit our willingness to be trans-*
> *formed?*
>
> *How can we help each other to live by the values of the Beatitudes?*

Blessed are those who are persecuted for righteousness' sake, for theirs is the kingdom of heaven.

PRAYERS

> *Almighty God,*
> *you have broken the tyranny of sin*
> *and have sent the Spirit of your Son into*
> *our hearts whereby we call you Father:*

give us grace to dedicate our freedom to your service,
that we and all creation may be brought
to the glorious liberty of the children of God;
through Jesus Christ your Son our Lord,
who is alive and reigns with you,
in the unity of the Holy Spirit,
one God, now and for ever. Amen
Collect for the 3rd Sunday after Trinity

Prevent us, O Lord, in all our doings
with thy most gracious favour, and
further us with thy continual help;
that in all our works, begun, continued,
and ended in thee, we may glorify
thy holy Name, and finally by thy
mercy obtain everlasting life;
through Jesus Christ our Lord. Amen
Communion Collect (BCP)

TWELVE

LIVING DIFFERENTLY

*Blessed is she who believed there would be a fulfilment
of what was spoken to her by the Lord.*

Standing back from our journey through each of the Beatitudes one overwhelming theme comes through. It is central to the life and teaching of Christ and is at the heart of the Beatitudes. It is the kingdom of God – the breaking in of God's generous, life-giving love, especially in the places of pain and brokenness in our world. Each pair of the Beatitudes uncovers important aspects of the vision that fired and sustained the remarkable life of Jesus Christ.

The kingdom is about being fully alive (poor in spirit and mourning) to the joys and struggles of life. The parables about seed growing secretly, the yeast in the dough, and the sower, highlight this inner vitality of God's presence. The kingdom of heaven comes, therefore, as a challenge to a culture which sees life in terms of consuming and looking for material satisfaction. It points rather to a life rooted in the soil of human frailty and open to the realm of the spirit. Life is really about living in openness as creatures before the Creator.

The kingdom is about yielding to another's agenda (meekness and a hunger for righteousness). This 'higher agenda' is graphically portrayed in parables such as the Prodigal Son and the Good Samaritan. It is demonstrated in the raising of the dead, and the healing of lepers, and the willingness of Christ to go the way of the cross. The kingdom of heaven comes, therefore, as a challenge to a culture which sees true freedom as being answerable to no one, having all you want and living for your own ends. It points rather to the essentially interdependent nature of human life and to the truth that even the nihilist philosopher Sartre recognized, that no one is happy unless they have a cause worth dying for. Life really is about seeking first the kingdom of God.

The kingdom is about generosity (mercy and pure in heart) as the heartbeat of the universe. Christ went about 'doing good', taught the power of forgiveness, gave welcome to outcasts and life to the poor, the sick and those on the margins of his world. The kingdom of heaven comes, therefore, as a challenge to an acquisitive culture, which with its abuse of the natural world and its resources, is in danger of 'dying of consumption'. It points rather to self-giving as the way to find ourselves. Life really is about sharing in God's generosity to all.

The kingdom is about love as the way to bring about change (peacemaking and persecution). In working for the coming of the kingdom in his own life, Christ was eager to bring wholeness wherever he went, even if hostility was the response to his upsetting of patterns of injustice. It took him to the cross and, in that ultimate experience of persecution, to bringing about the greatest work of peacemaking ever accomplished. It was the way of self-giving love. The kingdom of heaven comes, therefore, as a challenge to a culture which swings from opting out to hitting out. It points rather to the power of love and of non-violent forms of bringing about change. Life really is about learning to love with a love that comes from above.

But, though we see glimpses of this different way of living, we know it is a battle in our culture to hold on to this 'heavenly vision'.

THE BEATITUDES
These words are not just for Christians ... they are for the world,
and the future of the world depends on the extent
to which they are taken seriously and applied imaginatively.

Stuart Blanch, *The way of blessedness*

COMFORTABLE BRITAIN

An important reason for that struggle to stay true to Christ's vision for life, as expressed in these Beatitudes, is that the dynamic of Western society is one of addiction to comfort. The pursuit of material well-being is one of the most obvious evidences of this. Other marks include a preference for watching something on television rather than getting involved more directly, a dislike of any long-term commitment, an unwillingness to put ourselves out in the service of others and a reluctance to take risks.

What Christians tend to be slow in noticing is that *we are part of that society*. This strong commitment to personal freedom and personal comfort shapes the church's living, not just the culture around us. Middle England, as Bishop David Sheppard put it, is 'comfortable Britain'. The problem is that the church has often become too associated with that culture. The temptation is to practise a comfortable form of Christianity: one that makes few demands and avoids being distinct for fear of being thought different. The pressure is subtle but real. It is a pressure to conform to prevailing cultural norms, to settle for less. Some of the indications of this which I have observed in five years of travelling around the country are as follows.

A lowering of our sights from Christ to the church. I love the church and am deeply committed to it, but its only reason for existence is to be the community gathered around Christ and living out the good news of God's love for all creation which he brought into being. Yet often I have found people enthusiastic in maintaining a beautiful and historic building yet uncertain and tongue-tied when expressing the faith for which the building stands. The focus all too easily shifts from Jesus Christ and the coming of his kingdom to the keeping open of a particular building. These goals are by no means necessarily opposed to each other, but to put all the emphasis on the organization or building and little on the One in whose name it exists, is indeed a lowering of sights. It is the forgetting of our heritage under the guise of maintaining it.

A desire not to be thought different. Although our culture tends to knock traditions and norms and accepted patterns of behaviour, it is in fact a strongly conformist culture. Watch the children of any school where uniform has recently been abolished and you will see just how quickly a new 'uniform' emerges – often adding intense pressure on young people whose parents can ill afford the latest style of shoes or other 'gear'. Christians are too often eager to conform, wanting people to know that we are 'normal', can have 'fun' and are no different. Being different for the sake of it never was part of Christ's call; but being free to live by his values rather than the prevailing values in the culture around us is part of both our heritage and our calling. That vocation is to live in the culture in which we are placed and yet live by a distinct set of values which the Beatitudes highlight. Christ, in his incarnation, has shown us what is involved in being both deeply immersed in society yet living differently in it. He calls us to follow the same path in our setting in life.

A failure of nerve. There is much that is good in the way of generosity of living and hidden acts of love and service through the church. However, there is a certain failure of nerve evident in its life. This is not a call for a more strident or heart-on-the-sleeve form of Christianity, but rather a recognition that Christianity is essentially a way of life. It is something more than a Sunday habit, membership of a particular organization, or a private matter 'between me and my God'. The earliest term for the faith was the Way. The very survival of the church may rest on this recovery of a faith worth living, and dying, for; of a vision to inspire, direct and motivate us. That vision needs to be not simply a vision of what the church might be, but of what God desires for the whole of his creation.

For a church to be worth preserving
it needs to practise a religion that is extremely tough;
it needs to make spiritual demands and intellectual demands.

Michael de-la-Noy: *The Church of England, a portrait*

THE VISION OF SHALOM

A key concept that lay behind both Jesus' teaching about the kingdom and the nature of peace, and its frequent cost in persecution, is the Old Testament theme of *shalom. Shalom* is still today the way that Jews greet each other. But it is much more than a social greeting – our equivalent of 'hello'. It is, rather, a vision of a new order. Central to its meaning is the idea of balance. For the trapeze artist and the human body, the rain forest and an orchestra, dancing and the play of children, balance is foundational. *Shalom* is about the interplay of a number of forces which together bring about a living reality.

One of the biblical stories of *shalom* comes at the end of the story of Joseph and his turbulent relationship with his brothers. The fact that it comes at the end is itself significant, for *shalom* points us to the vision of what we long for but do not yet see. In the end, Joseph and his brothers do find this harmony, balance and joy – but not without cost and pain.

> Realizing that their father was dead, Joseph's brothers said, 'What if Joseph still bears a grudge against us and pays us back in full for all the wrong that we did to him?' So they approached Joseph, saying, 'Your father gave this instruction before he died, "Say to Joseph: I beg you, forgive the crime of your brothers and the wrong they did in harming you." Now therefore please forgive the crime of the servants of the God of your fathers.' Joseph wept when they spoke to him. Then his brothers wept, fell down before him, and said, 'We are here as your slaves.' But Joseph said to them, 'Do not be afraid. Am I in the place of God? Even though you intended to do harm to me, God intended it for good, in order to preserve a numerous people, as he is doing today. So have no fear; I myself will provide for you and your little ones.' In this way he reassured them, speaking kindly to them. (Genesis 50:15–21)

The brothers cannot believe they are forgiven, so try to control Joseph – yet again. But Joseph has learned, through painful experiences, not to hold onto bitterness but rather to live within a 'regime' of forgiveness. Because of this he can be a peacemaker. It involves real engagement with the gap between what he longs for (harmony, *shalom*) and what he sees his brothers expect (revenge). He minds the gap and is moved to tears. But he moves on, into the peacemaking that brings himself down to the right place ('Am I in the place of God?') and lifts his brothers up ('in this way he reassured them'). That reassurance is not just in words of forgiveness but in acts of kindness ('I myself will provide for you').

Shalom is a vision of harmony at every level. A vision of the lion and lamb lying down together, of the new Jerusalem, of the End Times, of the coming of the Messiah. That vision involves everyone having a part to play – to the full – and yet in so doing contributing to something that is bigger than any of the parts. It involves, like dance and play which are pictures of *shalom*, the interplay of form and freedom, structure and spontaneity.

The only remedy for the inevitability of history is forgiveness.

Hannah Arendt, Jewish philosopher

THE WAY OF LOVE

Wonderful though visions are, the fact remains that our biggest problem lies not in having them but in bringing them into being. How do we bring *shalom* into being in our world? The final pair of Beatitudes (peacemakers and the persecuted) point to a radically new way of bringing about change in a broken and divided world. It is the way of love, and of overcoming evil with good.

It is this that constitutes the 'new way' of Christ. It is the way of getting at the root without destroying that which you are addressing. Again, the surgeon's work is a picture of this process. By the strange method of putting the patient in a near-death situation (in other words, anaesthetized), then cutting open the body and removing the cause of disease (whatever is frustrating *shalom*, wholeness), the body is restored to wholeness.

Peacemaking also involves this life-through-death pattern of operating. It is essentially a pattern that respects the body, yet prunes to make whole and more fruitful. All too easily our instinct, when we see wrong, is to write off those who do wrong; we want to destroy organizations, and demolish the structure of the organization that oppresses us. We do this with ourselves, writing ourselves off as 'useless' and 'good for nothing'; we also take this destructive approach when we demonize groups who are in some way culturally different from others (from another race, sex, creed or culture). We do the same with governments and multinational corporations. Love, however, calls us to work like the surgeon, cutting out what is wrong so that the person, situation or organization is not destroyed but rathter restored to life and wholeness.

We find ourselves either wanting to drop the knife ('this is beyond me/us') or stick it in ('a curse on all your plans'). But Jesus has called us to another way. It is a way in which we become the knife, and our lives means of uncovering wrong, removing – often through the strange power of forgiveness – the obstacles to wholeness, and affirming that which we serve in all that is life-giving in its nature. Martin Luther King was a fine example of this when he confronted the racial injustices of his day. Rather than take up a position of hostility to white America he appealed to the soul of the nation. He spoke of the final frontier of freedom, of giving *all* Americans (black and white together) an equal share in the life and resources of the nation. He sought to build a vision big enough to embrace all. The 'rainbow people' image of South Africa similarly offers a vision that will count everyone in, value the sheer differences in the community, and make room for all.

This radical way of making peace sees that peace is a seamless robe stretching from the inner attitudes and motivations of individuals, their physical circumstances and personal stories, through to the way in which groups and organizations develop their own subtle yet powerful ways of defending themselves and making sure that power is in the hands of the few.

How we address injustice is as vital as *that* we address it. We can, with the wrong approach, simply add to the problems and multiply the injustices if we do not pay attention here. Look at many of the 'revolutions' in history and they are just that – things that go round without advancing. Typically in a revolution, what changes is who is doing the oppressing and who is being oppressed. Oppression as such is not removed: it just changes hands.

Jesus has shown us it is possible to address the harmful forces in us and in groups in a way that does deal with the underlying sickness and make for wholeness. It is essentially the way of love, of overcoming evil with good, well expressed by Paul when he wrote:

> Do not be overcome by evil, but overcome evil with good. (Romans 12:21)

It is striking that the very next verses address the attitude to the state (Romans 13). In them Paul urges respect for the structures of authority and describes them as 'instituted by God'. We can see just how true this is when lawful authority, even oppressive lawful authority, collapses in a country such as has happened in the recent past in the former state of Yugoslavia, and before that in Lebanon. Nobody gains by destroying the body, whether the human body, the body of an organization or the body politic of a country. Change can only come about – again as the surgeon shows us – when we love what we desire to change.

We become what we hate.

Walter Wink, *Engaging the powers*

CAN IT EVER WORK?

It might all seem too idealistic if it was not for the fact that some of the most striking expressions of this way have taken place in the last century of the second millennium. History may well identify the spread of peaceful means of addressing oppressive forces and systems as one of the great marks of the twentieth century. This is so despite the fact that more people have been killed in war in that same century than in all the preceding five thousand years of recorded history. Certainly we are living in the most devastatingly armed (or 'over-armed') culture in human history.

Yet there is another side that we too easily miss. From Gandhi in India to Lech Walesa in Poland, this has been a century of almost unprecedented change through peaceful means. Thirteen nations were involved in the dismantling of totalitarian regimes in 1989, including such vast power blocs as the Soviet Union itself and many of the East European states (Poland, East Germany, Hungary, Czechoslovakia, Bulgaria, Romania, Albania, Yugoslavia and more besides). South Africa has experienced a remarkable and substantial revolution, largely by peaceful means. Martin Luther King used, as noted above, the same approach in addressing racism in the USA. Rarely has the world seen so much change brought about by so little recourse to violence.

It is this strong passion to bring about peace by peaceful means which lay behind the sayings of Jesus that are so easily misunderstood:

You have heard it said, 'An eye for an eye and a tooth for a tooth.' But I say to you, Do not resist an evildoer. But if someone strikes you on the right cheek, turn the other also; and if anyone wants to sue you and take your coat, give your cloak as well; and if anyone forces you to go one mile, go also the second mile.' (Matthew 5:38–41)

Contrary to popular understanding this is not an encouragement to let people walk all over us, but rather an encouragement to look for creative ways of practising passive resistance. If a Roman soldier demanded, in Jesus' day, that you carry their belongings you were required to do so for one mile. Jesus is saying, 'Shame them into stopping this practice by carrying on the journey until they beg you to put the burden down.' Soldiers could be severely punished for having people carry their burden more than a mile. They would end up pleading to be given their load back – and perhaps wary of trying it again. Examples of the power of such an approach abound.

It is participation in these and other actions for peace in every area of life that is involved in the living out of our baptism into Christ's death and resurrection. Such costly peacemaking is in the baptismal job description of every follower of Christ.

THIRTEEN

INVITATION TO PILGRIMAGE

Blessed are those whose strength is in you,
who have set their hearts on pilgrimage.

Psalm 84:5, NIV

This study of the Beatitudes would not be complete without some final reflections on the ways in which they can help to shape and enrich the living-out of the Christian life, both by individuals and in churches, as well as through contributing the values that emerge from them to the world we live in.

We have seen that they not only describe the character and characteristics of the children of the kingdom, but give an outline of the journey of faith on which the disciple of Christ has embarked. They invite us to journey together with Christ into the kingdom. What follows is an exploration of various aspects of that journey. However, before doing so, it is good to see Christ's relationship to the Beatitudes as also being an expression of his pilgrimage through life.

THE PILGRIM CHRIST

The point was made in the Introduction that the life of Jesus Christ is the key which unlocks the Beatitudes. It is in Him that we see them lived out, and therefore rightly interpreted. The Beatitudes have been approached from this angle throughout our study. But there is a further way in which we can see Christ's living out these Beatitudes, for they seem to mark four significant phases, or emphases, in his life.

The first phase, of openness to God and to life, is seen in his early years, up to and including his baptism. He was eager to discover more when he went as a twelve-year-old to the Temple. He was eager for more of God through John's baptism. It is his openness to life that strikes us particularly in those early stages of his own life.

The second phase is one of eagerness to discover and do the will of his Father. He says exactly that in his temptations – that we live, are nourished, by every word that comes from God. We see him engaging in prayer, and quickly discerning what God is doing in each new situation. His first sermon at Nazareth is energized by this sense of discovery and vocation – which was there also in his baptism.

The third phase is one of merciful and discerning action. This is the phase of his healing and preaching ministry: the bulk of the recorded time of the gospel accounts. Jesus goes around 'doing good and healing all manner of sickness', being the 'friend of sinners' and 'speaking with authority'. Mercy, generosity, goodness are the central thrusts of Jesus' ministry.

The fourth phase is that of passion. Here Jesus goes to the fullest extent in being an agent of God's peace in a hostile, suspicious and unbelieving setting. Peacemaking, not least for Jerusalem, leads to the final showdown with the hostile forces, ending seemingly in the 'defeat' of the cross – which none the less turns out to be vindicated through the resurrection.

In so far as this is a valid interpretation of the Beatitudes as a map of the life of Christ, we need to guard against any idea that he stopped being open to God when he moved into generous living, or ceased to seek God's will once he engaged in peacemaking. All the Beatitudes apply all the time to Christ and his disciples. Nonetheless, there does seem to be a progression of emphasis through them.

So now we turn to some concluding thoughts about how the Beatitudes shape and enrich our living of the Christian life.

PRAYER AS JOURNEY

There are many ways to engage with the Beatitudes, but our starting point must be prayer. Here it is all too easy to get off on the wrong foot by praying in a way which negates all that the Beatitudes are saying to us. We wrong-foot ourselves whenever our prayer is filled with anxious pleading for gifts that are already ours; we would do better to rejoice in those gifts and receive them by faith. Similarly, the too frequent instinct to put ourselves down is not a good companion with the scriptures which constantly underline that we are blessed – valued, precious and loved by God. The Beatitudes are not a 'put-down'. They are a gift, a 'hand up' and a 'come-on'; as such they are an invitation to go this way through life.

Here are some of the steps that we can take on this pilgrimage of prayer through the Beatitudes.

Since the Beatitudes are in the first place a description of Christ, the right starting point is to use them as a pathway to *worship*. Just as a prism breaks up light into its constituent colours, so the Beatitudes reveal the many-sided nature of Christ. By using them rather like icons – pictures we see through to get at the truth they reveal – we give praise to God for Christ as the one who is truly poor in spirit, meek, pure, and so on. Seeing and using them as the basis for worship is also a wonderful antidote to any lingering sense of hearing them as a put-down.

The next step is to approach the Beatitudes with *thanksgiving*. They are to be received as gift, for they are a description of the inheritance of faith, of Christ's 'last will and testament'. This is why they stand at the head of the Sermon on the Mount. They describe the character of the children of the kingdom; and children can only live by the resources made available to them. The Beatitudes describe the generous 'settlement' God has made on those who have turned in faith to Christ. Thanksgiving is thus the best place to begin this process of reception of the Beatitudes. It is not easy, for we find it difficult to live by grace – but it is both our calling and our heritage.

A further stage is to see the Beatitudes as a framework for *personal prayer*. Just as the Lord's Prayer is a list of 'headings' under which we are to pray, so the Beatitudes can also work in this same way. The Meditations at the end of each chapter are designed to help in this way. Here in particular it is helpful to see the Beatitudes as a map of reality which helps us to plot both our present location and the direction we should choose to be going in. They are, therefore, ideally suited as a framework for personal review, reflection and 'assessment'. This personal application of the Beatitudes is likely to include specific petition as well as the practice of 'listening prayer' in which we seek to discern the call of God. The framework on pp. 180–181 is an outline for just such a use of the Beatitudes.

Another way of travelling through the Beatitudes is by using them as a framework for *intercession*. This in itself is an act of mercy, purity and blessing. It is simply a matter of remembering before God those known to us who at present are poor in spirit, mourning, hungering after righteousness. It is a very simple way of praying for others.

In all the above the assumption is that prayer is approached *meditatively*. We do this by reflecting on the rich diversity of ways in which Jesus and the saints of scripture and the church have lived out the Beatitudes. This meditative approach is also needed in seeking to discern how they speak to us today. Meditation has been described as rather like sucking a boiled sweet. The aim is not to bite it and consume it in a moment. Rather the art is in gently moving the texts around our mind, letting them refreshing our thinking and praying. It is a 'slow release' method of prayer. In the frantic culture in which most of us live, that in itself can be healing to the soul.

HEARING THE BEATITUDES

The meditative use of the Beatitudes highlights another way in which they can guide our path through life. They can be used not only as a framework with which to address God in prayer, but also as a way in which God speaks to us. The very act of studying them allows this to happen. There are also further steps we can take to enhance our hearing what God communicates to us through these sayings of Jesus. They are as follows.

Seeing them as gift. It has been argued throughout this book that this is how we should allow the Beatitudes to speak to and nourish us. We can do this not only in prayer but in the midst of everyday life. Are we aware of our need for strength, wisdom and help from beyond ourselves? Then, in listening to being poor in spirit, we can still ourselves – in a moment, just by a shift of attitude – and be open to what God desires to give us. Meekness and humility require that we look for the answer to come through other human beings and through our daily circumstances, not just in some narrowly 'religious' way. Are we irritated by family or those with

Praying through the Beatitudes

A guide to using the Beatitudes as a framework for intercession:

◆ *poor in spirit*

What are the resources for living that God has given me for which I can give thanks?

Where am I, at present, aware of needing grace, help, wisdom? Bring that before God, with open hands to receive the answers to our prayers.

◆ *mourning*

Where am I aware of a gap between what is and what God desires?

Seek to be in touch with any sadness or anger about the brokenness in our life, and in the whole world. Work with, rather than run from, the pain we feel.

◆ *meekness*

Where do we lack wisdom to know the will of God or find His grace making a difference?

Are there ways in which we are anxiously 'fixing the world after our own wisdom'? In that case we need to yield to God's timing, direction and purposes.

◆ *hungering and thirsting after righteousness*

What are the real longings of our heart? Dare to be honest to God!

Are there ways in which God desires to affirm, evangelize or strengthen these desires?

Are there concerns for his purposes that I need to be open to which are not part of my thinking or living as yet?

◆ *merciful*

Where, not least in relation to the things identified under 'mourning', is God calling me to give away the mercy and grace I have received?

Are there enemies, people I would rather not think of right now, on whom I can pray God's blessing?

◆ *pure in heart*

Where do I need fresh vision, and the ability to see through to the heart of what is going on in this situation?

Where does my own attitude need 'evangelizing' into God's discerning purity?

◆ *peacemakers*

Where, in areas that I can influence, is God wanting to bring wholeness into being?

Where, in the area simply of my concern, is God calling me, through that 'burden' to pray for the coming of peace?

Might there be a contribution I can make beyond prayer?

◆ *persecution*

What are the ways in which I experience temptation or pressure to move off the pathway of the Beatitudes? Receive God's strength to keep on the Way.

whom we work? Then, taking our stand on the gift of mercy, we can look for ways of seeing things from the perspective of other people. Does the injustice that others are experiencing stir up anger within us? Then, recognizing that we are called and gifted for peacemaking (not necessarily because of our temperament but by grace), we can look to see what positive contribution for good we could make in that situation.

Here are resources to draw on in the whole of our living. They tell us the good news that we are not shut up to our own abilities and resources. Allowing the Beatitudes to speak to us in this way can be a deeply refreshing way of engaging with them. This approach is wonderfully expressed by the Psalmist:

Blessed are those whose strength is in you,
who have set their hearts on pilgrimage,
Who going through the valley of dryness
find there springs from which to drink:
till the autumn rain shall clothe it with blessings.
They go from strength to strength:
they appear every one of them
before the God of gods in Zion. (Psalm 84:5–7)[1]

Here indeed is a living well to refresh us on our pilgrimage through life.

Hearing them as vocation. If faith is a journey, then the Beatitudes are the signposts. At the critical points on the journey we can listen to them telling us where we are and where we should be going. If life has been particularly fraught, then the stillness involved in owning that we are poor in spirit can calm us down and help us

1 Verse 5, NIV, verses 6–7 ASB Psalms.

see the gap that has opened up between our programme and the will of God. If we are caught in a situation where we cannot see what can be done, then we are likely – by the very experience – to be hearing a call to hunger and thirst after righteousness. If we find ourselves at home, at church, at work, caught in a host of unresolved conflicts, then the call to peacemaking can help us discern the direction in which our contribution can be made. The key to hearing is letting the Beatitudes speak to us, address us and shape the direction we take in life.

Understand them as choices. The Beatitudes are not primarily descriptions of blessed *states*, but of holy *choices* we make in response to life. As such they address us as *vocations*. But vocations only have value if they are lived. To hear the call of God brings with it a call to choose that way. Indeed the root meaning of the words 'listen' and 'obey' is the same. Properly to hear is to obey. So recognizing in the Beatitudes a set of callings which address us through life can allow them to shape our living in surprising and unexpected ways. Poverty of spirit is a call to choose openness to God and others; meekness a call to submit our plans to the light of God's higher agenda. Purity of heart is a call to choose God's way of seeing life and others. Handling the Beatitudes as choices allows them to shape who we are.

SHARING IN THE BEATITUDES

God has been revealed to us as Trinity. That means that God is community – a community of love. The Christian understands that the fullest expression of the image of God in human beings is therefore through our 'dwelling together in love'.

If the Beatitudes really are to shape our lifestyle, provide us with a set of values by which to live, and reveal the goodness of

God in the process, then we will need others to help us. Indeed it is in the mutual help – and coping with the moments of mutual un helpfulness which are a part of any relationship – that we discover their relevance and power to shape us.

This means that studying the Beatitudes, and this book, in a group is one of the best ways of engaging with them. Such study is greatly enriched where there is a conscious commitment to develop a shared way of life. In a culture shaped by individualism and the consumer mentality, we need a group of people around us who can help us – and whom we can assist in helping – to order our lives around the things that really matter. We need others to achieve this. So finding others willing to share that venture with us is one of the best things we can do.

Once a group has worked through the Beatitudes they will need to identify the four themes which they see as best expressing the message of these texts to them. They then need to decide how to set about helping each other to live out these truths. It may be helpful for such groups to keep in mind a checklist such as the following one to help them in the outworking of a shared way of life.

- what steps have we taken to *give expression* to each/any of these themes?
- what *encouragements* have we had along the way?
- what *problems* and *answers* have we discovered in the practice of these truths?
- what are the *next steps* we can take to live out any of these themes?
- how can we *share* these insights and steps with those we live and work with?

In this way a simple 'rule of life' or – better – 'way of life' can be built up and used as a compass to help us make progress on the way of the Beatitudes.

Such groups may well be set up by the local church, or be a new way of handling existing groups. But we do not need to wait for that. Any group of believers, not least those who work together or have other interests in common, can form cells of the kingdom seeking to explore and live out the Beatitudes.

What such groups will need to do is recognize that becoming such a cell will require persistence, honesty, a willingness to face and overcome obstacles and, above all, a willingness to allow the Beatitudes to have a significant – even if unpredictable – effect on our lifestyle. A group whose only commitment is spending time to study these scriptures, but who are insulating themselves from any willingness to share in their outworking, are likely to find that their study bears a meagre harvest.

IT IS ALL DONE BY GRACE

Whatever else happens, it is vital that in taking the Beatitudes seriously we do not take ourselves too seriously. The key word in them all is *Blessed* and it should point us continually to God's grace. They need first to be embraced with *joy*, because the One who most fully lived these truths has entrusted them to us and promised to make them a reality in our own experience.

So in all our engagement with the Beatitudes, we need to recognize that any 'success' in living them out is done by grace. This means that *thankfulness* for what we have received through them is the necessary starting point, the best means of travelling through them, and our true destination.

Particularly if we are doing so in the company of others, we need to affirm our own *liberty* to do what we judge to be right without needing to be proved right, and without any pressure to conform. We need also to fight for the freedom of others to be at liberty in their response to these scriptures.

Holding on to our *security* as children of God, as those who have already been gifted in Christ with the marks of the these Beatitudes, is also important. They are neither an exam nor a reward for good behaviour. They are a *gift* to be opened and enjoyed and wondered at and a vocation to be listened to and followed, because we are already members of the family.

Seeing the Beatitudes also as gifts that we are to give to others is another way in which grace is rightly expressed. They are good gifts to scatter liberally around our path through life.

God's purpose is that in our embracing these glorious insights we will find them to be a means of grace; a living well to refresh us. That purpose is also that through these few words, in a world searching for values that make sense of life, we might discover and show God's way for all humanity to be living well.

LIST OF SOURCES

p.xiii, p.51, p.151 Michael Crosby, *Spirituality of the Beatitudes*. Orbis Books, Maryknoll, New York, 1992.

p.xvi Michael Crosby, *House of disciples*. Orbis Books, Maryknoll, New York, 1988.

p.xix John Stott, *Christian counter-culture*. Inter-Varsity Press, Leicester, 1978.

p.6, p.92, p.109, p.154 Simon Tugwell, *The Beatitudes*. Darton, Longman and Todd, London, 1980.

p.8 Henri Nouwen, *Life of the Beloved*. Hodder and Stoughton, London, 1992.

p.10 John Bradshaw, *Healing the shame that binds you*. Health Communications Inc, Florida, 1988.

p.11 Luke Johnson, *Sharing possessions*. SCM Press, London, 1986.

p.20 Gerard Broccolo, *Vital spiritualities*. Ave Maria Press, Indiana, 1990.

p.24 Dietrich Bonhoeffer.

p.26, p.150 Kathy Galloway, *Struggles to love*. SPCK, London, 1994.

p.33 J. Neville Ward, *Five for sorrow, ten for joy*. Darton, Longman and Todd, London, 1993.

p.36 C. S. Lewis, *Prayer: Letters to Malcolm*, Collins, Fontana Books, London, 1964.

p.38 Jean-Pierre de Caussade, *Self-abandonment to divine providence*. Collins, Fontana Library of Theology and Philosophy, London, 1972.

p.40 Terry Waite, *Taken on trust*. Hodder and Stoughton, London, 1993.

p.49 A. T. Pierson, *George Müller of Bristol*. Quoted by Stuart Blanch in *The way of blessedness*. Hodder and Stoughton, London, 1985.

p.53 Stephen Covey, *The seven habits of highly effective people*. Simon and Schuster, London, 1992.

p.65 Duchrow and Liedke, *Shalom*. WCC Publications, Geneva, 1987.

p.69 Leanne Payne, *Healing presence*. Crossway Books, Illinois, 1989.

p.76 Mother Teresa of Calcutta.

p.78 John Baillie, *Our knowledge of God*. Oxford University Press, London, 1939.

p.79 James Philip, *Christian maturity*. Inter-Varsity Fellowship, London, 1964.

p.81 Forrester/McDonald/Tellini, *Encounter with God*. T & T Clark, Edinburgh, 1983.

p.93 Robin Greenwood, *Practising community*. SPCK, London, 1996.

p.96 Edwin Markham.

p.99 C. S. Lewis, 'The weight of glory', *Screwtape proposes a toast*, Fontana Books, London, 1965.

p.106 Kathleen Raine, *Collected Poems*. Hamish Hamilton, London, 1956.

p.111 Origen. Quoted by Stuart Blanch in *The way of blessedness*. Hodder and Stoughton, London, 1985.

p.120 David Bosch, *Transforming mission*. Orbis Books, Maryknoll, New York, 1992.

p.124 Jean-Jacques Suurmond, *Word and Spirit at play*. SCM Press, London, 1994.

p.126 John F. Kavanaugh, *Still following Christ in a consumer society*. Orbis Books, Maryknoll, New York, 1991.

p.130, p.135 *Debt cutters handbook*. Jubilee 2000, London, 1996.

p.154 Alexander Schmemann, *Great Lent*. St. Vladimir's Seminary Press, USA, 1974.

p.158 Diarmuid O'Murchu, *Reclaiming spirituality*. Gill and Macmillan, Dublin, 1997.

p.165 Stuart Blanch, *The way of blessedness*. Hodder and Stoughton, London, 1985.

p.167 Michael de-la-Noy, *The Church of England, a portrait*. Simon and Schuster, London, 1993.

p.169 Hannah Arendt, Jewish philosopher. Quoted in *Bringing the olive branch*, Beulah Wood, World Vision UK, Milton Keynes, 1996.

p.172 Walter Wink, *Engaging the powers*. Fortress Press, Minneapolis, 1992.

ACKNOWLEDGEMENTS

The following publishers have kindly given permission for the reprinting of copyright material:

The extracts from 'Will you come and follow me?' by John L. Bell and Graham Maule on pp. 13, 58 and 144 are from the *Heaven shall not wait* collection and are used by permission of the Iona Community. Copyright © 1987 WGRG Iona Community, Glasgow G51 3UU.

The extract from 'Kyrie eleison' by Jodi Page Clark on p. 29 is used by permission of Kingsway's Thankyou Music. Copyright © 1976 Celebration Services/Kingsway's Thankyou Music, PO Box 75, Eastbourne, East Sussex BN23 6NW.

The extract from 'Meekness and majesty' by Graham Kendrick on pp. 57–58 is used by permission of Kingsway's Thankyou Music. Copyright © 1986 Kingsway's Thankyou Music, PO Box 75, Eastbourne, East Sussex BN23 6NW.

The extract from 'He who would valiant be' by Percy Dearmer (1867–1936), after John Bunyan on p. 160 is used by permission of Oxford University Press.